HIGH PERFORMANCE
BEAUTY

Makeup & Skin Care for
Dance, Cheer, Show Choir,
Pageants & Ice Skating

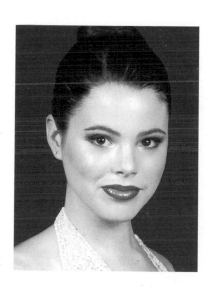

CHRISTINE DION

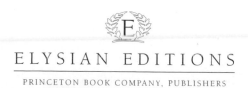

ELYSIAN EDITIONS

PRINCETON BOOK COMPANY, PUBLISHERS

Important: The material presented in this manual is for general education purposes only. It is not intended as a substitute for specific medical advice. Medical advice can be obtained only from a qualified and reliable doctor.

The author and publisher assume no responsibility or liability for any consequences of the failure of the reader to obtain such specific medical advice from a qualified doctor or dermatologist, nor for any or all of the information contained in this book.

In case of poor skin health we strongly advise the reader to consult a qualified doctor.

Cover design, text design and composition by Elizabeth Helmetsie

Copyright ©2007 by Elysian Editions
An imprint of Princeton Book Company, Publishers
614 Route 130, Hightstown, NJ 08520

Library of Congress Cataloging-in-Publication Data

Dion, Christine.
  High performance beauty: makeup & skin care for dance, cheer, show choir, pageants
  & ice skating/Christine Dion.
    p. : (chiefly color) ; cm.
  ISBN–13: 978–0–87127–303–1
  ISBN–10: 0–87127–303–9
  1. Theatrical makeup—Handbooks, manuals, etc. 2. Skin—Care and hygiene.
  3. Entertainers—Health and hygiene. I. Title.
  PN2068 .D56 2007
                                              792.027

Printed in Korea   2 3 4 5 6 7 8 9

Contents

With thanks to

Neil McGovern for his endless support, hours of help and a lifetime of encouragement.

Sherri Mardones and Tilden Patterson for beautiful photography.

All my fabulous and perfect models who, with no experience in front of the camera, posed like cover girls and acted like pros.

The wonderful costume companies who brought these looks to life:
Upstage, JD Designs, Lathers, Class Act, Retter World, All Star Challenge Spirit Wear and America's Best Spirit Wear

My publisher, Princeton Book Company, for their excitement, vision and guidance in bringing this helpful book into the industry we all love.

Introduction

Performers, whether they are dancers, cheerleaders, ice skaters or show choir members, combine strength and beauty through music and movement. No matter the age or size of these powerful, yet graceful athletes, they have a lovely radiance that comes from within. Performers are a celebration of expression and form. They are art in movement. Makeup enhances and helps express the beauty that is already in motion.

Makeup is an art form, and before an artist can paint a masterpiece it is important to prepare the canvas…your face! This key beauty factor is often forgotten when creating a beautiful makeup look. Performers have special skin care needs. As truly athletes in makeup, heat, perspiration and excess oil can create problems like bumps, pimples, blackheads and irritation. Having a deep understanding of skin, your skin's type, how to care for it and how to prevent problems from occurring will keep your looks in top condition. Learning nature's healing secrets will keep you glowing on the outside and healthy on the inside. Good skin is the perfect canvas for flawless makeup.

Your looks are more than just your face. Hair care, body care and the steps to keep your looks in top condition are an important part of life for any busy performer. Dancers, cheerleaders and other athletic performers express their craft with their bodies. When the body is the focus so is the skin. Good grooming, hygiene and following beauty advice for smooth, glowing skin will give you extra body confidence. Remember with all that time on stage, it's important to take some time off. Make maintaining beautiful skin a part of your life. Learn how to relax, soothe tired muscles and heal rough, callused feet. Taking time for a little at-home spa using natural herbs, aromatherapy and color therapy makes relaxing, healing and rejuvenating fun.

Performers love makeup, shimmer and glitter. They love to show personality and to add drama. Remember that stage light is very different from daylight—and color choices, especially foundation color, is very important. In daylight mistakes are easily noticed. For rehearsals, auditions, interviews, performing outdoors or just for the stage of life, makeup should be toned down to show your natural beauty by defining your features and adding radiance. Understanding how to choose the right foundation for your skin type and undertone, as well as how to use color to accent your hair, eyes and skin will keep your looks flawless in the brightest outdoor light.

A professional photograph, the headshot, is the calling card of any serious performer, and knowing how to apply natural-looking photography makeup is key. Achieving a photo-perfect look will help you stand out as a pro.

Good makeup artistry is not only choosing the right colors, but knowing how to enhance your features. I call the technique of using makeup to sculpt and correct your features to perfection "Face Physics." This is truly where the art of makeup comes into play. There are many ways to use color, shading and highlighting. This knowledge will perfect your application and will be useful from street makeup to the strongest large stage performance face. The tools, including brushes and their care, are all necessary to enable the artist to create a real masterpiece. Understanding how to use his or her tools is essential for every artist.

With a strong understanding of makeup application, you're ready to paint the high performance face for stage light. This includes performances on both small to large stages, even stadiums. I've taken the guesswork out of choosing colors to make it easy for you.

Consider the age of the performer. Application for a junior is lighter than the look for an adult or teen. Deep skin tones will need stronger color pigments and men will need just enough to create masculine good looks. In this book, I emphasize these differences to help you avoid embarrassing mistakes. Performance makeup requires a little more thought and technique, especially when using extras like white pencils, false lashes, glitter and rhinestones. Those extras really create show appeal and dazzle your audience. With a little practice you'll have the moves down in no time. Of course, before any show, a makeup-look rehearsal is always a good idea.

This book is a collection of the techniques and tips—they work!—that I have enjoyed passing on to performers through my beauty columns and workshops. It combines the answers to all the questions asked by my readers, performers, their mothers, coaches and instructors. I hope this book makes the challenging and expressive task of makeup application easier. May you find as much enjoyment doing your own makeup as I have found doing yours.

To My Readers

You have arrived in the spotlight. Your dedication, discipline and effort to rise above the ordinary have made you extraordinary. Along with recognition comes responsibility that goes beyond the stage. Others now take notice of your style, charisma and talent; you stand out. Bring the passion and confidence felt on stage into everything you do. Be an inspiration to all who know you. The more you respect and honor yourself as well as others, the more radiance you create and the more beautiful you become. Take pride in your appearance. Make your personal best a lifestyle. Love and appreciate your body, express your spirit with joy and shine like the star you are.

Best of wishes,
Christine Dion

1
Skin Care

Before any artist begins to paint a masterpiece, she first prepares the canvas. Your skin is the canvas for your makeup. Smooth, healthy skin is a must for a flawless makeup application. Here is how to get in step with the right skin care moves.

Everybody has skin care challenges from time to time, but performers have more than most. Performers really give their skin a workout! What can you do to get your skin in shape? In the following chapters, we present an in-depth focus on face, hair and body care. Uncover beauty secrets using botanical treatments, at-home pampering tips and healthy-skin foods to keep you and your skin in top condition.

Why skin care before makeup is important

We know that perspiration not only creates a makeup meltdown, but can also cause a multitude of skin problems. The wrong skin care routine and makeup formula only make things worse. Hormones, diet and stress have an effect on your skin health too.

Skin must be cleansed and hydrated before any makeup is applied. When skin is not properly hydrated, moisture is pulled out of makeup foundation, causing it to fade. Dehydrated skin will produce more oil to compensate for dryness. This excess oil will cause your foundation to fall apart and run. Good skin care, including a light oil-free moisturizer, creates a perfect canvas to hold makeup and keep you looking fresh.

First, it helps to understand your skin. Skin is your body's largest organ. From the top of your head to the tips of your toes, you are covered in this protective marvel.

Skin is made up of two layers, the *epidermis* and the *dermis*. Within each of these layers are several other layers. To keep it simple, we will discuss only the most important layers.

The epidermis is the surface skin, made up of many layers of skin cells. The bottom layer of the epidermis is the *basal* layer, where *melanin* is produced. Melanin gives your skin its color. Sun exposure increases the amount of melanin produced in your skin. This is called a suntan. A tan is the basal layer's response to damage from the sun as it tries to repair and protect your skin. **Always use sunscreen to avoid damage!** Signs of extreme damage are brown spots, white spots, freckles, irritation and, of course, skin cancer. (See more about sunscreens on page 19.) The basal layer is also where skin cells are born. Their health depends on the nutrients and oxygen carried to them by blood vessels.

Blood vessels originate in the deepest group of layers, the dermis. The dermis layer also contains oil glands, sweat glands and fat cells. Collagen is the "bio glue" that holds it all together. It gives your skin elasticity and strength. Sun, stress, poor diet, pollution and age break down collagen which causes your skin to wrinkle and sag after time.

Oil Glands, Pimples, Blackheads, Whiteheads & Cysts

Oil glands are located in the dermis, right next to the hair follicle. They produce oil (known as *sebum*) that covers the skin and locks water in. This keeps your skin smooth and soft. Yes, oil is a good thing! Oil protects and locks in existing water, but remember, the only way to get water there is to drink it. That's why it is important to drink eight glasses of water a day—or more if you are doing intense workouts.

Sweat glands increase oil production. When perspiration mixes with bacteria and oil, it can cause little bumps and irritations on the skin.

When dead skin cells fall down into a hair follicle shaft it becomes blocked. Bacteria are a big problem because they often live on dead skin cells and can cause an infection in the pore. Oil and white blood cells (to fight bacteria) can build up and cause swelling. This is a pimple, a blockage deep in the pore.

Blackheads and whiteheads are also blockages close to the surface of the skin. Since oil reaches the surface of your skin through pores, it is important to keep these pores as free from bacteria and dead skin as possible. If a pore opening becomes blocked at the surface, a blackhead or a whitehead will develop.

This is where *exfoliation*, or removing dead skin cells, comes in. Would you believe that a large portion of household dust is your own dead skin cells? Well, it is! Humans shed their skin all the time. As dead skin cells are shed from your body, new skin cells produced in the basal layer replace them. Problems can occur when a number of dead skin cells remains on your skin and mix with bacteria, causing breakouts. You can exfoliate by using a clean washcloth when cleansing, a gentle facial scrub, buff puff, or natural acids like *salicylic acid* products. (More information will follow later in this chapter.)

A cyst is a deep, painful bump on the skin. The outer walls of the hair follicle, weakened deep in the epidermis by the existence of a pimple, break open. The contents leak into the dermis causing inflammation. White blood cells (pus) form and a red, round hard bump appears. These are best left alone to heal, or see a dermatologist for treatment.

Back acne can result from hair conditioner residue. Be sure to thoroughly rinse conditioner out of your hair and off your skin. Perspiration can contribute to this problem so wear cotton clothing when perspiring. A back brush with antibacterial body wash can help keep the area clean and clear. Be sure to keep the back brush in a ventilated area to avoid bacteria build-up. Use an antibacterial astringent containing salicylic acid in a small spray bottle—to more easily reach your back.

Preventing Breakouts & Breakout Treatment

You will find many treatments to dry out pimples at drug stores and cosmetic counters. These are spot remedies which attack only the surface of the skin. Since pimples begin to form weeks before you ever see them, the key is to treat the skin **before** the breakout. Look for daily treatment products containing *benzyl peroxide* to kill bacteria, slough off dead skin cells and control sebum production; *salicylic acids* to unplug and clear pores; or *sulfur* to reduce redness and swelling. *Neosporin*® antibiotic ointment helps reduce redness.

Squeezing pimples can result in scarring. To help extract a pimple (only if it has a white top), place a warm, clean washcloth over the area and massage gently. If the pimple bursts, sterilize the area with an antibacterial astringent. Try to do this at night so the pimple has time to heal. Makeup can be irritating and cause infection.

A dermatologist can prescribe a topical antibacterial treatment if breakouts continue.

How to avoid bacteria and other pimple-causing enemies

- Keep your skin clean. Wash your face in the morning, before rehearsal and at night before sleep. **Never** go to sleep with your makeup on. Your skin rejuvenates itself at night—makeup interferes with this process.

- Use products on your face that were formulated for the face (not the body) and for your skin type.

- Use clean washcloths and buff puffs. Change everyday.

- Anything that touches your face should be clean, including your hands! Fingernails are filled with bacteria. Avoid scratching and touching face with hands, fingers or nails. Once a week, wash your brushes, puffs and sponges with a cleanser like dish washing liquid to remove bacteria.

- Clean your phone and rims of eyeglasses with rubbing alcohol.

- Do not share someone else's products.

- Keep hair, including bangs, off your face. Styling products like hair spray, gel or mousse can irritate and clog pores. Other products to avoid on facial skin are Vaseline, baby oil, lipstick and gloss.

- Use oil-free makeup and moisturizers.

- Be careful when using eyelash glue to apply rhinestones and oily gel glitter on your face. Never use gloss or Vaseline.

- Pillowcases can contribute to rashes and breakouts. Harsh detergents, especially those used in many hotels, can be irritating to sensitive skin. Bring your own pillowcase for performances out of town. Wash pillowcases, and all linens and towels, at home once a week.

Oil and water

Our skin can be both oily and dry. Some people have oily skin with a dry surface. Many have dry surface skin due to harsh products used to dry the oil. This skin type should try an oil-free moisturizer. Since dead skin can sometimes be confused with dry skin, exfoliation is important to keep skin smooth, free of flakes and tiny bumps.

Those with dry skin have less water deep in the skin layers and don't produce enough oil to hold it in. Moisturizers containing a little oil are best for this skin type. Remember, the skin produces perspiration and oil when you are performing. Even people with dry skin should consider oil-free products when working strenuously during practice or performance.

Determining Your Skin Type

It is not always easy to know your skin type. Here is a description of skin types and their characteristics to help you. Allow skin 20 minutes to respond after cleansing in order to best identify your skin type. (However, only a dermatologist can positively identify your skin type.)

Oily

Shortly after cleansing, your skin becomes oily and shiny. You often have breakouts. Your skin feels heavy, making you want to clean it more than twice a day. Pores are enlarged and may have black or whiteheads.

Normal to oily

Skin can become oily in specific areas like the forehead, nose and chin. You may have some breakouts or find you break out once a month. Your skin may feel oily in some areas and dry or normal in others. In the winter months you are drier and in the summer months more oily. Pore size is small to medium.

Normal

Skin may have a small amount of oil. You rarely have breakouts. A pink glow exists from good circulation. There may be a few blackheads and pore size is small to medium.

Normal to dry

Skin feels normal, except for dry areas like the cheeks or forehead. In the winter you feel tight and dry after cleansing and in the summer you feel normal. You never get breakouts. Pores are small without blackheads.

Dry

Your skin feels tight after cleansing, and you feel that you need to moisturize right away. It is flaky at times and can feel uncomfortable and tight in harsh weather. Generally you look dry and never get breakouts. Pores are small or invisible. Body skin may be very dry and chaps easily.

Sensitive

Sensitive skin is not common. Poor skin care, including the wrong products for your skin type, stress, diet, harsh weather and overexposure to the sun may all contribute to irritated, problematic skin. If you have been prone to rashes and red, itchy irritations in the past, then you probably have sensitive skin. This skin type can be very sensitive to food. Eat foods like organic whole grains, fruits and vegetables that do not cause inflammation. Stay away from refined carbohydrates, sugary or starchy processed foods.

If you suddenly develop an irritation, here are a few things to check out:

- Have you been outdoors and have a sunburn or windburn? If so, use an appropriate treatment and try to avoid severe weather.

- Have you recently started using a new product? If so, stop using it and see if it clears up. Always read and follow the instructions provided with your skin care products.

- Other possible irritants to look for are preservatives in cosmetics, mineral oil, lanolin, petrolatum, certain fragrances, dyes, old makeup, dirty brushes, paba (para-aminobenzoic acid) or titanium dioxide (both found in sunscreens) and pollution.

Remember:

- Most people with sensitive skin are allergic to some fabrics. (A dermatologist can test your skin for allergies.)

- If you are using a new product line, test one item at a time. Do a patch test—put the product on your forearm for several days in a row to see if you develop a reaction.

- Look for words on the product label like "allergy tested," "fragrance free," "all natural," "hypo-allergenic," "dermatologist tested," "unscented," or "non-comedogenic" for breakouts; "ophthalmologist tested" for eyes.

Healthy Skin Comes from Mind, Body & Spirit

Your skin is not just a separate, individual organ. It is connected to the rest of your body. Your emotions, what you eat and the stress you put on your body greatly affect the condition of your skin.

Learn to take it easy on yourself emotionally. Get rid of guilt, fear, anxiety, tension and stress. An example of a response to emotion is the way skin becomes flushed from embarrassment, perspires when nervous or becomes oily when under stress. Just beneath the surface, nerve cells actually touch your dermis. Nervousness or stress can act as a stimulus to many skin disorders like hives, eczema, psoriasis, acne and rosacea. Hormones, diets full of processed foods, fast food, sugar, caffeine, salt, and fats, as well as hard exercise, can create a strain on your system. A body out of balance will exhibit dry skin that is oily at the same time, breakouts, rashes, premature wrinkles, puffy eyes, oily hair and dandruff.

On the bright side, love and joy can improve your skin and give you a beautiful glow.

TIP

Drink at least eight glasses of water a day, eat lots of fresh fruits and vegetables and find the time for relaxation.

Daily Routine & Products

When you develop a daily routine, use common sense. If your skin doesn't react well to a routine or product, change it! No one knows your skin better than you do, so use your own experience to develop a skin care routine. When in doubt, consult a qualified medical doctor. Always read product labels.

Most of the products you buy for your routine care will be labeled for oily, normal, dry or a range (i.e. normal to dry or normal to oily). Always start by choosing the product that best fits, or is closest to, your type.

The use of exfoliating acid products is popular today. Exfoliating acids are called alpha hydroxy, glycolic, salicylic (best for breakouts), or multi-hydroxy acids. These acids are found in many face cleansers, toners, astringents and moisturizers. When used daily they break down dead skin, which is then easily removed during cleansing. A weekly scrub will buff off dead skin build-up. Acid products can be very effective but can also increase sun sensitivity by thinning the surface layer of your skin. Always use a sunscreen with these products.

Cleansing your face

For oily skin, start with products like antibacterial gel or lotion cleansers. Gels and products that foam when you use them are good for removing excess oil, but hard to use on the go. Lotion washes are more gentle and good for oily to normal skin types. Experiment to see what works best for you. If you are a dry skin type

7

TIPS

The amount of poduct to use when washing your face is about the size of a nickel.

Using too much toner can cause patchy dry areas on the skin, especially around the nose and mouth. In the middle of a cotton square, use an amount the size of a quarter.

To avoid using too much cream, use an amount about the size of a dime for face and throat.

Gently pat the eye treatment on with your ring finger. Never rub the delicate eye tissue. If you use it at night, try not to get too close to the eyes as it could cause swelling and irritation.

you may want to use a lotion or a cream cleanser. These are gentle and contain moisturizers so that dry skin feels more comfortable after cleansing. Cleansers come in a variety of creams, gels, lotions or bars. Choose the one that is best for you and, of course, made for facial skin use.

Makeup remover

An average facial cleanser can't remove a lot of makeup. If you are wearing a full face of makeup or heavy foundation, you may want to try a makeup remover before cleansing. A great makeup remover is almond oil, massaged over the face, then removed with a moist cotton pad. Never wipe away makeup with a tissue: tissue paper is made of fine wood shavings that can scratch and irritate skin. Washing your face twice and following with a toner or astringent can work to remove most makeup.

Use non-oily eye makeup remover pads to remove mascara and eye shadow. Waterproof mascara will need to be removed by an oily eye makeup remover. Avoid baby oil or Vaseline as they are difficult to break down by washing and can leave a film on the eyes. Be sure to whisk away eye makeup in downward strokes, not side to side, as product can cause eye irritation. Never use soap around your eyes.

Toners and astringents

Toners and astringents are liquids that help condition, restore pH levels (the balance of alkalinity and acidity in your body) and remove any leftover debris from your skin. Many astringents for oily skin types may contain alcohol, which can dry the surface of skin. For healthier natural ingredients, look for alchohol-free astringents that use strong herbs to kill bacteria and control oil.

Dry skin types should choose products called toners or fresheners. These are usually alcohol-free and less drying. Use with a cotton pad (100% cotton) and don't forget your hairline (the hairline can develop pimples and is often missed when cleansing). Avoid your eye area, as it is very sensitive and easily damaged. Again, don't forget to read product labels!

Moisturizers

Oil-free moisturizers in gel or lotion formulas are best for oily to normal skin types. For normal to dry skin, use a lotion containing a little natural oil. Dry skin types should use a cream formula because they contain more oil, are richer and feel more comfortable. Listen to your skin. It is not uncommon to use a lighter formula in the summer and a heavier formula in the winter as needed. All skin types should use oil-free formulas when performing because perspiration increases the production of oil.

Don't forget your eye area, as it is the first to get wrinkles! Moisturizers for the eye area are creams, lotions or gels specifically designed for that area. They should not be used on the face as they are too concentrated. Use as needed.

Daytime is the most important time to use an eye treatment because environmental exposure and squinting can damage the delicate eye area and cause premature aging. Avoid using a facial moisturizer around the eyes—they are not designed for that area and can cause puffiness.

TLC: Special Treatments & Products

Scrubs

Scrubs help to exfoliate (remove dead skin) and are beneficial for a healthy complexion. Scrubs should be used as often as needed or as directed by the product instructions. Please note that when you first start using a scrub your skin may actually breakout even more than usual. Don't freak out! When you gently remove dead skin with a scrub, the circulation improves. The oil in your skin is now free to flow from the pores and is no longer blocked by the dead skin cells. Breakouts that were brewing and have not yet reached the surface can do so all at once. It takes two weeks to get on track; be patient.

The best scrubs for the skin should be made from either smooth nonabrasive grains or from the meat of nuts, like almond meal, not the shell of the nut or pit of a fruit that is jagged and abrasive. Oatmeal is another very gentle exfoliant. Using a clean washcloth with your facial cleanser every day is a great way to exfoliate, too. Some people like buff puffs for exfoliating. These can be harsh to the skin. Use them gently and not every day.

Do not use a scrub on open pimples—it can spread the infection. Scrubs are great for blackheads and tiny bumps. Remember to avoid your eyes.

Masks

Clay masks: Clay has long been valued for its earthy minerals and botanical benefits. It absorbs oil, removes dead skin and helps with whiteheads and blackheads. Clay increases circulation and can leave your skin looking flushed after it is removed. Clay masks, because they remove oil, are usually for oily skin. Most oily skin types will probably want to use a clay mask twice a month. Typically, clay masks are nonirritating and should only be left on ten minutes, at most. It is best not to allow clay to dry thoroughly. Apply clay thickly, like frosting on a cake, so it will take longer to dry. And, as with all products, stop using it if any irritation occurs.

Moisturizing masks: This kind of mask is for dry to normal skin; however, dehydrated oily skin can benefit from these as well. Moisture masks infuse moisture into the skin, calm, soothe and help increase circulation.

Peel-off masks moisturize and remove dead skin. If you are prone to breakouts, you should avoid peel-off masks because they can leave behind residues that clog your pores.

- Use masks according to the current condition of your skin. For instance, if you have normally dry skin, yet feel especially oily, you may want to use a clay mask rather than a moisturizing mask.

- Masks should be used from once or twice a week to once a month. It is up to you to judge when you need a mask and what type.

- When using a mask always make sure your face is clean and patted dry before application. It should be applied smoothly, evenly and fairly thickly, so that no skin can be seen beneath it. Avoid the areas around your eyes and lips! Clay in the eyebrows is especially difficult to wash off.

- While wearing a mask, remember that you are pampering yourself. Take it easy, put your feet up, listen to some music and relax; you deserve it. One of the best places to wear a mask is in a luxurious bath. Add a hydrating and soothing bath treatment. While you soak the steam will prevent your mask from drying out too fast. The time for yourself will do wonders for your complexion and your body, as well as reduce stress. And you know that reducing stress helps stops blemishes, too.

Nature's Gift to Our Skin: Botanical Beauty Treatments

The benefits of herbs and at-home natural treatments

TIP

Try growing herbs at home. It's fun!

Herbal home remedies of the past are still beneficial for today's skin care. Some of the ingredients found in the latest skin care products are good enough to eat; they smell great, too.

There are many herbal skin care products on the market including those that I produce. They contain many of the herbs listed below. Natural products are definitely worth a look as your skin absorbs everything—and sends it right into your body. Staying away from products filled with chemicals can only be a good thing. As our skin absorbs these natural products, oil and toxins are pushed out through the pores. That's why it is so important to allow the skin to breathe. Products with petrolatum, like Vaseline and mineral oil (baby oil is mostly mineral oil), cut off the skin's ability to breathe and can be harmful in the long run. Healthy products are as important as a healthy diet. Skin care products filled with vitamins, minerals, fruit, vegetable and botanical extracts not only make you feel

Herbs to the Rescue

TO CLEAR, REGULATE & INCREASE CIRCULATION IN THE SKIN

Try products with rosemary, eucalyptus, sage, thyme, spearmint, lavender, yarrow, tea tree oil and ivy. They are often used in toners and can greatly benefit oily skin.

FOR FIRMER AND YOUNGER-LOOKING SKIN

Try products with chamomile (which also calms the body) and rose hip seed oil (moisturizes and protects). Cornflower extract reduces facial lines and will firm the skin.

TO INCREASE CIRCULATION & GIVE SKIN A HEALTHY GLOW

Try products with orchid (also a moisture retainer), peppermint, mint, lavender and ginseng. Oolong tea and green tea reduce under eye puffiness.

TO SOOTHE & CALM THE SKIN, & REMOVE REDNESS & IRRITATION

Try products with aloe vera (which also moistens), marigold, St. John's wort (also helps with chapping), witch hazel (a mild astringent), linden tree and camphor tree, licorice (it desensitizes), chamomile, kola nut and wild pansy.

TO MOISTURIZE & KEEP SKIN SOFT

Try products with Irish moss, violet (for cleansing), marshmallow, comfrey and jojoba oil (the closest natural oil to our own sebum). Cold pressed and extra virgin oils such as olive, almond, coconut (anti-bacterial too), avocado and grape seed are wonderful.

DULL SKIN

Dull skin lacks water, not oil. Symptoms can range from lack of vibrancy to tiny pimples and patchy red, dry and itchy skin. Helpful herbs to look for are marine extracts, citrus or lactic acids and plant extracts like chamomile, sage or rosemary.

DRY SKIN

Dry skin lacks water and oil. Symptoms include thin, tight, cracked, flaky skin. This skin type needs a moisturizer that really penetrates. Helpful herbs to look for are rosewater, aloe vera and products containing glycerin.

OILY SKIN

Oily skin secretes too much oil, breaks out and shows large pores. Helpful herbs to look for are clarifying sage, mint, pine, camphor, rosemary, tea tree oil, watercress and eucalyptus.

Remember, if you are not used to taking good care of your skin (as is recommended here) and using regular treatments, you may notice a sudden increase in breakouts after a new regime has been started. Do not get discouraged! After this initial break-out condition your skin should improve dramatically.

To avoid puffy eyes, avoid salty foods because they cause water retention. At night, sleep in a room with good fresh-air circulation (to prevent allergies); put an extra pillow under your head while sleeping (it keeps swelling from the face); keep face creams away from your eye area.

great but bring health and vitality. Try to read labels and really learn how product ingredients, including herbs, affect your skin. Don't apply an herb essence or oil directly to your skin—make sure it's diluted in a cream or oil formula.

At-home masks

It's fun to take time for a little pampering—and if it can be with all-natural ingredients that are healthy for your skin and body—it's even better! Our grandmothers knew these methods, now you can use them too.

We want to remind you that before using any of these treatments it is helpful to consult a qualified doctor (dermatologists are specialists in treating the skin). If you are allergic to any treatment, do not use it; try something different.

Do not apply at-home masks and facials to irritated skin as they may aggravate the problem. Use masks as soon as you prepare them—they can spoil.

To purify and remove dead skin, try this tropical treatment to give your skin a glow: blend together half a papaya, one teaspoon of honey and one teaspoon of lime or lemon juice. Apply to face. Leave on eight to twelve minutes, then rinse. For a fast treatment, take the meaty part of a papaya peel and rub gently on your face. Leave on for five to eight minutes.

For a super moisturizer try this avocado boost: Mash a ripe avocado and apply it to your skin. Leave on a few minutes and then rinse. It helps relieve red, rough skin, too. For dry, patchy areas, puree one peeled mashed banana and one tablespoon of olive oil. Leave on twenty minutes, then rinse. To soothe irritated skin, dip a cloth in cool milk or buttermilk and let it rest on your face for fifteen minutes, then rinse with cold water. Plain yogurt massaged into skin or aloe vera gel works great, too.

At-home beauty treatments

- To restore skin to its proper pH (acid/alkaline) balance, stir one-half teaspoon of apple cider vinegar in eight ounces of water. Apply to face and throat using cotton pads in upward sweeping strokes.

- To break down heavy makeup, massage natural cold-pressed avocado, olive, almond or coconut oil over the skin. Remove with cotton pads saturated with water. Then cleanse skin.

- To treat a cold, place a few drops of eucalyptus oil in a bowl of hot water. With a towel over your head, breathe in the healing oils. This will clear mucus and helps you to breathe.

- For puffy eyes—hold the bowl part of a chilled spoon over each eye, or place two moist, cool chamomile tea bags over your eyes for five to ten minutes. (Brown tea bags work well, too.) Chilled cucumber slices placed on your eyes for about ten minutes will reduce swelling and whiten eyes. Another secret, popular with models, is to refrigerate your eye moisturizer. When the cold eye cream or gel is applied it can quickly reduce puffiness.

Aromatherapy & the Power of Steam

Aromatherapy is treatment with scent. Different aromas are thought to have different effects on us physically as well as on our moods and feelings. Some invigorate (citrus or mint, for example), some help us relax (like lavender or chamomile), some make us feel nostalgic (rose and sandalwood) and some relieve nausea or headaches (chamomile or spearmint). The list goes on and on.

Aromatherapy can be very effective not only because it can treat your mind, but also can treat your skin at the same time with natural healers. Steaming is a great way to release this healing power. When boiling water is poured over the natural healers, the oils are released into the steam and are absorbed into your skin as well as breathed into your body.

A Wonderful Spa-like Skin Steam

Make sure your face is clean and makeup free.

Use a peel-off mask or a scrub (as needed) to remove dead skin cells. This insures that your pores are clear as they open during steaming.

Combine a handful of each: fresh mint or peppermint, lavender, chamomile, rosehips (the center bud of the rose) and a few orange or lemon peels. Use tea bags of these ingredients if you can't get them fresh.

Place the mixture in a large bowl.

Fill the bowl a little over half full with hot water.

Cover your head with a towel, put your face over the bowl, breathe in and steam for about five minutes.

Splash your face with cool water.

Follow with your favorite facial treatment like a clay or moisturizing mask, if needed, and rinse. With the pores open, this is a perfect time to use your mask.

Rinse with warm water or use a warm washcloth to remove mask.

Moisturize face and eyes as well as feet and hands.

Now relax!

How to quench a thirsty body and skin

The most important fluid in your body is water, and it needs a lot of it—up to a gallon a day! The best water to drink is natural spring water, bottled at the source. Purified or distilled water is a fine second choice, but try to avoid tap water because of its added chemicals. Shaking your bottled water a few times helps oxygenate it for faster absorption into the body. Place a slice of lemon in each glass of water to help your body quickly absorb the moisture and regain balance. A slice of cucumber is wonderful addition, too. Used at many top spas, a slice of cucumber in your glass will cleanse and refresh the body.

Use water to restore dehydrated facial skin: place chamomile or rose hips tea bags into a small spray bottle filled with spring water. Mist your face a few times a day. Try green tea, it has powerful skin antioxidants and provides natural sun protection. Misting is especially helpful in dry climates or during air travel.

Restore Lost Fluids with Food

Fruits such as strawberries, all melons (especially cantaloupe), tomatoes, grapes, oranges, kiwis, apples, pineapples and grapefruit help restore fluids and provide healthy vitamins, too.

Restore fluids with this great quenching cocktail

Pour boiling water into a pot of fresh mint leaves or mint tea bags, then cool. Put ice in a glass and fill half the glass with tea. Fill the rest of the glass with sparkling mineral water or seltzer. Sweeten with honey or organic pure white grape juice.

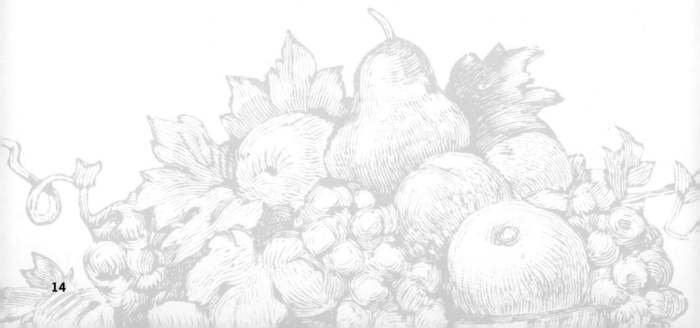

Beautiful Skin From What You Eat & Drink

Here is a list of natural additives like fruits, vegetables, vitamins and minerals found in the latest skin care products and the magical effect they have on your skin. Many of these can be taken orally as supplements, as well:

Vitamin E protects against damage from ultraviolet light and the ozone that is produced when sunlight meets car exhaust and other pollutants. Helps to repair damage to the upper layer of skin and works as a moisturizer by preventing evaporation of water from the skin cells. As a supplement it repairs and protects cells.

Vitamin C protects against environmental damage and stress. Look for *Ester* C. As a supplement, Ester C helps skin form collagen, increases support and elasticity and nurtures capillaries that supply blood to your skin. It also builds stronger teeth.

Vitamin A increases elasticity and thickness of the skin. It helps normalize dry skin. It helps to reverse damage from environmental exposure. It adds luster to your hair and a glow to skin. As a supplement, it helps skin retain moisture and fights acne.

Beta-carotene is a powerful antioxidant. It helps protect skin from aging due to environmental exposure and stress.

Pro-vitamin B5 works as a natural moisturizer for the skin, hair, and nails. It has a healing effect on the skin. As a supplement B vitamins improve nerve health.

Pro-vitamin D5 enhances vitamin D levels in the skin, which decreases as we age. As a supplement it is vital for bone health.

Tomatoes can be a powerful antioxidant, helping to restore and heal skin. When eaten, they work as an antioxidant for fighting cancer.

Carrot oil protects skin from environmental damage, heals and smoothes dry skin.

Oolong tea, white tea and green tea help increase circulation, reduce puffiness and contains antioxydants. Drinking tea helps in the same way. Green tea has been known to reduce pain from exercise, lower blood sugar and reduce the risk of cancer.

Ginger is a skin and muscle stimulant. It increases circulation. When eaten or sipped in tea, it calms stomach upset and reduces inflammation.

The minerals zinc, copper, iron, magnesium, silver and gold all improve the skin's ability to function, eliminate toxins, increase circulation and help the renewal of cells. Find the same results when taken as a supplement.

Other skin vitamins include alpha lipoic acid, which protects healthy cells and helps retain moisture; hyrolonic acid, which builds collagen and muscle tone;

omega 3 to build our immune system and to slow the aging process; and selenium (taken with vitamin E) prevents cellular damage. *Note:* Follow the recommended daily allowances for vitamins and minerals since too much of some vitamins and minerals can cause health problems.

Foods that enhance beauty

Food is fuel for your body. Every time you put food in your mouth, ask, "What is this going to do for me?" If you do not understand what is important for your health and what is harmful, begin the quest for knowledge now. Be sure to eat a variety of natural, chemical-free foods. Your body needs a balance of carbohydrates, fats, protein, vitamins, minerals and water to stay healthy. Research has shown that organic vegetables and fruits contain more vitamins and are free from dangerous chemicals used in the growing process and in the preparation of the soil. Whenever possible, choose organically grown produce. Your body is the most important possession you have! Treasure it and respect your health. Here are a few tips to get you started:

Eat Breakfast!

THE BEAUTY SHAKE

1/2 cup organic plain yogurt
one cup frozen berries
two cups water
one teaspoon blackstrap molasses
one scoop whey protein powder
one banana
one teaspoon flaxseed oil

Blend and drink to your health. *Note:* Blackstrap molasses is filled with minerals like iron, copper, calcium, manganese and potassium. It tastes sweet without calories.

THE BEAUTY BREAKFAST

On the stovetop (not the microwave) cook steel cut Irish oatmeal. When it is done, stir in one teaspoon of flaxseed oil, top with sliced apples and almonds and sprinkle with a little cinnamon and finish with skim milk. For a change, try rice milk instead of cow's milk. All these ingredients will insure better health, beautiful skin and a perfect start to your day.

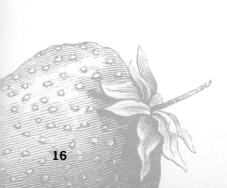
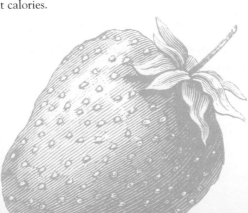

Healthy skin foods—Vegetables, especially tomatoes, celery, carrots, corn, winter squash, alfalfa sprouts, cucumber, broccoli, squash, yams, onions, ginger, garlic, red peppers and pumpkin seeds. Fruits like berries (especially blueberries), apples, pomegranates, cranberries, watermelon, cantaloupe, citrus fruits like oranges and grapefruit, mangoes, papaya, guava, kiwi and grapes. Nuts such as almonds, macadamias, peanuts and walnuts make a wonderful snack and their oils greatly benefit your skin. Be sure to eat nuts that are raw and not toasted or fried. Store them in the refrigerator.

Salt—Use sea salt that has natural minerals. Too much processed salt can strain your system, causing cellulite and water retention.

Meat—If you must eat red meat, eat free range, grass-fed cattle that have not been given hormones or antibiotics. Focus on chicken (free range without hormones or antibiotics) and fish. Salmon, tuna, herring and sardines are filled with omega 3, a powerful antioxidant that builds beautiful skin. Salmon that is farm raised has had coloring added to create a pinkish hue to the meat. If you must eat farm-raised salmon, get it dye free.

Sugar—Sugar increases the aging process by breaking down collagen and causing sagging. Try natural sugar substitutes. Stay away from artificial sweeteners—they are filled with chemicals that attack the weakest part of the body causing damage and throwing your body out of balance.

Flour—Avoid white flour and empty carbohydrates. Eat foods made with wheat flour and natural grains.

Beverages—Soft drinks and diet sodas have no nutritional value. Drink tea, a natural antioxidant and healer, or organic unsweetened fruit juices. Try fruit juice mixed with natural sparkling water in place of soda. Water is the most important beverage of all!

Oils—Fried foods destroy the skin. Avoid hydrogenated oils, corn and vegetable oils. Use cold-processed virgin oils like olive, coconut, almond, sesame or grape seed oils. Flaxseed oil has omega 3 (like that in fish) and can be added cold to salads and oatmeal. When eating salads, add a little fat either from the oils listed here or from nuts and avocados. The fats help you better absorb the vitamins.

Soy—Be cautious when you eat soy products. Too much soy can increase estrogen in your body, can put hormones out of balance, negatively affect the thyroid and irritate digestion. Tofu has been fermented, so does not have this effect.

Yogurt—Sweetened yogurt has extremely high sugar content. Nonfat, organic plain yogurt mixed with fruit and blended into a shake or a smoothie is wonderful for digestion, boosts the immune system and provides calcium. To add natural sweetness use honey, agave nectar (an organic sweetener) or stevia (an herb that is sweeter than sugar) found at your local grocer or heath food store.

TIPS

For a wonderful healthy dessert, eat dark chocolate. Dark chocolate (at least 60% cocoa) is a wonderful antioxidant to slow aging and makes you feel good too!

Avoid the microwave when you can. Studies have shown that the plastics and metals used in microwave food containers leak into the food during the cooking process. Remove foods from their containers into glass or ceramic dishes before cooking in the microwave. Of course, it's always best to eat fresh foods whenever possible.

Dangers to Your Skin

The sun

Most skin damage comes from the sun. Those who wear SPF (sun protection factor) sunscreen of fifteen and up, who sit in the shade and wear a hat for protection, will greatly lower their risk of sun spots, liver spots, skin cancer and photo aging (the premature aging of the skin, wrinkles and sagging).

The sun isn't what it used to be. While it's true that the sun heals the skin and provides us with vitamin D, both of which are beneficial, we can get our daily requirement with about fifteen minutes, or less, of exposure a day. Let's face it: the sun's rays combined with chemicals in our atmosphere and the diminished ozone layer make the sun dangerous. Don't think tanning beds are safe either. Their harmful rays are even more damaging and increase the risk of skin cancer.

Because of the power of the sun these days, tanning and exposure to the sun have become a very dangerous and unhealthy fashion. Sun damage done today may not show up until ten to fifteen years later. Sun damage at age fifteen can result in aged, sun damaged skin at age twenty-five!

If you must be in the sun, then at least follow these steps, for better protection from exposure:

- Always use sunscreen. If you are prone to breakouts, oil-free sunscreen is available. (There are no excuses!)

- Wear a hat and good sunglasses (eyes can be damaged too) when outside. Don't forget your lips, which protrude and catch all the rays. Wearing lip gloss or shiny lipstick can be just like wearing oil on your skin, creating certain sunburn. Always wear a lipstick or balm containing a sunscreen if you plan a day out in the sun.

- Self-tanning lotions make you look tan but are not sun-safe. Your best bet is to tan with a self-tanner with the highest SPF sunscreen possible. Don't forget to reapply sunscreen as often as indicated.

- Always take a cover-up or a T-shirt with you. When you feel you have had enough, cover up exposed areas. Watch for arms and back of neck.

- Keep your sunscreen bottle in the shade. The bottle absorbs the sunlight and breaks down the sunscreen, making it ineffective.

- Never shave or wax your legs and bikini area the same day you are heading out to the beach or pool. Sun exposure, salt water, and chlorine can irritate your skin. Those nasty red bumps will appear. Even underarms can become irritated.

- Performers should be extra-careful to avoid tan lines. These are hard to cover up and can ruin the look of a costume.

What is a tan and how to ID your SPF

SPF means *sun protection factor*. An SPF of 15 means that you can spend fifteen times longer in the sun than you could without any protection. (SPF 20 means twenty times longer, and so on . . .)

- To figure out the SPF you need, first decide how long you are going to be in the sun. Then figure out how long it takes your skin to begin to burn. Divide your burn time into your exposure time, and that equals the SPF strength needed. If you really want to play it safe, double or even triple that figure.

- Time of day is important in your calculation as well. The sun is strongest during midday ("prime sun time"). Water (lakes, pools and oceans) and sand reflect the sun's rays, so even if you are in the shade you can still get sunburned.

- Most oils provide zero protection. They may actually encourage a burn.

- Note: We said a burn, not a tan. A tan comes from the production of melanin in your skin, protecting it from burning when exposed to the sun. I can't state it more clearly: **You cannot get a suntan unless you are being damaged by the sun!**

- The sun's rays are divided into three types:
  1) UVA rays penetrate into the connective tissue and are present wherever there is sunlight. They cause skin cancer, premature aging, wrinkles and sagging.
  2) UVB rays are present when the sun is strongest. They penetrate into the deepest cell layers and cause sunburn and blistering. Does not pass through glass.
  3) Infrared rays are heat rays, and the most damaging; they can even harm inner body organs. They are most effective when the sun is strongest.

Healthy skin is suntan-free skin. Protect yourself.

Watch out for these skin enemies

Cigarette smoke (yours and others) impairs the circulation in your skin and its ability to heal itself. Studies have shown that it takes twice as long to heal the skin of a smoker as that of a nonsmoker. Don't smoke! It is not only bad for the skin, but it is also horrible for the rest of your body.

Pollution can be incredibly harmful by disturbing the skin's natural pH balance and weakening its natural defenses. The solid particles in pollution adhere to your skin and can cause irritation and/or acne. Chemicals are all around us. Household products, plastics, paint and even carpeting contain chemicals that have shown to be toxic to the body.

Sun, cigarettes, chemicals and pollution can produce *free radicals*. Free radicals are unstable molecules that damage a healthy cell, causing the skin to break down—kind of like an apple becoming rotten. Our immune system fights them off, but if there are too many of them it just can't keep up. Reduce exposure whenever possible.

Drugs and alcohol are extremely taxing to the skin. They dehydrate and destroy healthy cells. Wanting beautiful skin is a great reason not to drink or take drugs.

Sugary or artificially sweetened sodas put strain on your body, causing your skin and body to become out of balance.

Fried foods have very little nutritional value. When oil is cooked to a temperature hot enough to fry foods, it turns into *trans fat*. Trans fatty acids are a type of unsaturated fat industrially created by partial hydrogenation of plant oils and animal fats and linked to chronic bad health conditions. It is very bad stuff!

Indoor heating can also dry out your skin. If you use a humidifier in your room at night, some specialists believe it is even better for your skin than a moisturizer.

To sum up: care & prevention tips

- Always use sunscreen. Use it on your face, neck and tops of hands (to avoid brown spots). Apply ten to fifteen minutes before going out (follow the directions). Be aware that sun damage can come through car windows as well as home windows.

- Make sure your sun products, including sunglasses, carry both UVA and UVB protection. Some antibiotics, medications and fragrances (especially citrus scents) can make you more sun sensitive.

- Avoid pulling and tugging at the skin on your face, especially around your eyes. When resting, avoid stretching your skin while lying on your face.

- Don't frown or raise your eyebrows and stop other face-wrinkling habits.

- Your skin repairs itself at night, so rest is vital. Never sleep in your makeup.

- Allow your skin to breathe. Go a day without makeup at least once a week.

- You already know this, but pass it on. Exercise increases blood circulation and rids your body of toxins through perspiration. Exercise at least thirty to forty-five minutes three times a week. It will also help you control stress.

- Apply facial moisturizers gently in upward strokes. Be extra-careful around your eyes and when removing makeup.

- Nothing ages you like stress. Take care of yourself, relax, enjoy quiet moments.

- Protect and exfoliate your lips.

- No drugs, sodas, alcohol or smoking.

- Regularly eat healthy foods for skin and body.

- As with everything in your life, "If it doesn't feel right, don't do it." In other words, you know subconsciously what you and your body need and don't need. Listen to your body!

- Keep makeup brushes clean (wash at least once a month) and powder puffs fresh. Throw out old makeup.

- Take care of your teeth, both for health and beauty. There's nothing like a great smile.

Skin Care Terms

This helpful list of terms found on packages and labels will make product shopping and finding the right products much easier:

Active ingredient—The ingredient that directly responds to an ailment or symptom, one that prevents a particular occurrence or is directed toward a desirable goal.

Allergy tested—A higher level of testing than *Dermatologist Tested*.

Dermatologist tested—At least one dermatologist has checked it out.

Organic—It usually means that the product does not contain any synthetic chemical ingredient or has been grown without chemicals. It contains, for example, no preservatives, artificial fragrance or dyes.

Collagen—Collagen is the skin's underlying structure. It provides both form and strength to the skin.

Silicones—Minerals that have the ability to repel water. They are sometimes used in formulating creams for holding better to the skin.

Superfatted soap—Soap rich in fat and oils designed for dry skin cleansing.

Exfoliate—To remove dead surface cells.

Fragrance free—No fragrance is used in the product.

Hypo-allergenic—Formulated to lower your chance of having an allergic reaction, although there are no Federal standards or definitions that govern the use of the term.

Humectant—A product that pulls in moisture from the air.

Non-comedegenic—The product should not irritate or clog pores.

Unscented—There is no scent in the product; however, a fragrance may be used to cover up or nullify a distasteful fragrance that naturally occurs in the product.

Always double check and read the ingredients on the labels for your protection.

A Beauty Note

Beautiful skin takes time. A great smile and a beautiful personality can improve your looks and keep you radiant every bit as much as beautiful skin does.

2
Hair, Body & Nail Care

Your facial skin care routine will keep your good looks in shape for years to come, but there is more to good looks than just your lovely face. The skin on your body has special needs and so does your hair. True beauty comes from looking radiant from head to toe.

Facial skin is thin and delicate. Body skin is much thicker and more prone to dehydration. Products used on the body are very different from those we use on the delicate skin of our face. Stress and exercise can create challenges to the appearance of body skin.

Body Care

With so much time on, you need time out. Performers love to keep on the move but sometimes your body says "*enough!*" Treat yourself to some tender loving care. Take time to take it easy and relax with these stress relief ideas for beautiful all-over skin.

Get your beauty sleep

One of the most important beauty treatments you can give your skin is getting at least seven to nine hours of sleep every night. While you sleep your skin uses this time to heal and rejuvenate. For better comfort, sleep with firm, fairly thick pillows that keep your head and neck from drooping toward the mattress. Polyester-filled pillows may work best, since foam doesn't stay in one place and down can compress. If you sleep on your side, put a pillow between your knees for support. So many ailments, including poor skin and body health, can be aggravated from the lack of a proper night's rest.

Shower-power for beautiful smooth skin

With easy at-home pampering, your skin will be soft, smooth, shiny and radiant in no time at all. The best time to bathe, shower or do any at-home body treatment is just before going to bed. Heat from the bath or shower brings your body temperature up. When you finish, your body cools down. This creates a relaxed, even sleepy, effect. It's not the best time to get dressed, run for the door, out to a busy day!

For a smooth skin shower treatment, begin with a clean rough sponge or washcloth filled with your favorite bath and shower gel. Scented body scrubs are also great and easy to use. Do a good all-over scrub, called exfoliation, to remove dead skin and increase circulation. This is the time to shave your legs. (See *Body hair, beware!* page 24.) Towel-dry your skin by patting, not rubbing, to leave skin slightly moist.

Follow with a rich herbal moisturizer of lavender, chamomile or almond (that soothes) or with ginger, mint, citrus or rosemary (that invigorates) to ease muscles.

Instead of a moisture cream or lotion, try cold pressed and organic oil, one of the best treatments for dry skin. The best oils combined or used alone are olive, sweet almond, avocado, coconut (a natural anti-bacterial), grape seed, sunflower and jojoba oils. They can be found at your local grocery or health food store. Before drying with a towel, apply oil liberally over dry areas like legs and arms while you are still in the shower. Oil seals in moisture, keeping skin smooth and silky. Apply to feet first, working up the legs toward your heart. (Avoid the bottoms of your feet so that you won't slip.) Hydrating your body from the feet up helps increase circulation, which removes toxins and strain. Towel dry, avoiding areas where oil has been applied so it has time to seal in moisture. This takes five to ten minutes.

Take the time to do this treatment at least twice a week to increase circulation and buff your skin to a smooth, radiant glow.

Hot on your feet

Tired, throbbing tootsies deserve some time off. First, soak your feet in warm water with your favorite mint bath gel to invigorate, or add cinnamon sticks to help feet smell fresh. A good foot soak not only soothes tired feet, but also softens skin for easy removal of calluses with a pumice stone. After the soak, use a pumice stone or foot file on rough spots, then hydrate with a rich, mint foot cream. A foot cream containing peppermint is cooling and soothing for worn-out feet. Don't forget to use footpads to protect the heels, as well as corn cushions and foot odor eaters.

Aching legs: take ten to kick back

Here's how to restore your legs and your serenity: turn on soothing music and turn down the lights. Massage your feet with a cream or oil, pressing gently across the bottoms of your feet. For best results, learn more about the tremendous healing powers in the soles of your feet from an ancient healing practice called *reflexology*. Essential oils (found at health food stores) containing ginger or rosemary can be mixed into your massage oil or cream to increase circulation. After massaging your feet, lie on your back, head flat, and elevate your feet with a few pillows under your ankles. Close your eyes and take deep breaths. This alters the circulation pattern, provides relief and relaxation and will give your face a little glow. Do this for at least ten minutes. *Absorbine Jr.*® has a really strong smell, but this penetrating roll-on ointment really can bring fast relief for aching muscles and hot, itchy feet.

Healthy legs

The key to beautiful healthy legs is a healthy diet, regular exercise and good circulation. Cellulite, the appearance of lumpy fat deposits under the skin, can accumulate where circulation is cut off. Avoid crossing your legs, and when hydrating legs, really massage them to get circulation moving. Limit your intake of carbonated diet sodas, processed, fried or frozen foods, caffeine, salt, soy sauce, white bread, muffins, cream, cheese or butter.

Body hair beware! Tips on unwanted hair

Performers expose a lot of skin. Hair removal is part of creating a clean, smooth look to the skin. Extensive exercise creates moisture and irritation, so make sure to wax or shave sensitive spots the day before a big workout or performance to avoid inflammation and little red bumps.

A good scrub before shaving helps to stimulate hairs for a closer shave. Make sure to use a double-blade razor for less irritation and shaving cream for easier glide. Sensitive areas will be less irritated if you shave in the direction the hair grows. Always apply an antibacterial astringent or a product specifically designed for use on those sensitive areas to help prevent red bumps and ingrown hairs. A bonus for removing unwanted hair, especially under the arms, is the reduction in body odor. Less hair means less chance of odor-causing bacteria to build up. Never use an old, dull razor. The life of an average razor is about eight uses.

Your At-home Spa

ONE

In the shower, wash and rinse your hair. Apply a deep conditioning or hot oil treatment and put on a shower cap.

TWO

Apply a clay mask to your face, throat and chest, avoiding eye area and brows. If your skin is very dry, apply a moisture mask to these areas instead.

THREE

Run a bath with hot water and add a beautiful herbal bath soak. To make an aromatic, soothing and healing bath soak, use one teaspoon each of botanicals such as sage, eucalyptus, lemon grass, lemon oil, rosemary and peppermint. Wrap them in a 5" x 5' cheesecloth bag and tie at the top. Toss the bag into the hot bath and breathe in the botanicals as they melt your stress away. Other aromatherapy bathing botanicals are mint, rose petals, lavender, chamomile and orange peel.

Bath salts are wonderful for easing muscles and removing toxins from skin. Mix them into your bath with the botanicals for an extra benefit.

FOUR

Light candles in the bathroom and play calm music or nature sounds. Close your eyes and let the steam from the bath, filled with the healing botanicals, relax you. The steam also prevents the your clay mask from drying out, so the minerals in the mask have time to soak into the skin. Soak no more than ten minutes. When finished, drain tub and shower, removing the hair conditioner and mask.

FIVE

Next, use an exfoliant (body scrub, sponge, clean washcloth or brush) and scrub away dead skin. This really gets the circulation flowing all over your body (especially arms and legs). Remember bath sponges and brushes should be left to air out in a dry place to avoid bacteria build-up. Sponges can be machine washed weekly with clothes.

SIX

Moisturize your entire body with rich moisture cream or body oil. Start at the feet and work up the legs toward the heart for increased circulation. Remember to moisturize when your skin is still wet so the moisturizer can seal in the skin's moisture. Your lotion will last longer too.

SEVEN

For sweet dreams, spray your pillow and bed sheets with a floral mist. A scent in lavender or rose is a good, soothing choice. Lie down and relax. Close your eyes and breathe deeply. Sweet dreams.

Short on time but high on stress? Try the *mini-spa*. Follow steps 1 and 2, then soak in the tub with bath oil. Make sure to pour bath oil in the tub *after* you get into the bath. Bath oil can lock in moisture on the skin only after your skin is already wet. If you step into a bath with oil already in it, the oil floating on the surface will stick to the skin and feel greasy. Go to steps 4 and 5, then to step 7 and relax.

The best way to control odor and perspiration

Since we are on the subject of odor, let's clear the air, so to speak, on questions I'm often asked. First, know the difference between deodorant and antiperspirant:

Deodorant does not fight perspiration, but does control odor with an antibacterial additive. Some deodorants are scented. These are best if you perspire very little.

Antiperspirant is a good choice if you perspire a lot. It reduces the flow of sweat with astringent salts.

Antiperspirant/deodorant combines the best of both and is ideal for performers who need both benefits. Try natural deodorants without aluminum.

A spot check: Underarm stains on fabrics can happen even with the best protection. They appear when the active ingredient in a sweat-controlling product combines with the skin's sebum (oil) to form a substance that water alone can't wash out. To remove, apply a liquid dry-cleaning solvent (available at drug stores), then a bit of clear dishwashing liquid and scrub with your fingers. Rinse thoroughly with warm water, repeating until the stain is gone. Wash the garment as the label recommends.

Soaking it up with botanicals

Here is all you need to know about the bath, how hot, what to put in, and how long to soak:

Muscle warm-up
Try a ten-minute warm bath (95° F–105° F) to increase the internal temperature of the muscles. This makes them more flexible and pliable which reduces the chance of injury.

Frazzled nerves
Try a ten to twenty minute bath in hot water (102°–104° F) that will dilate your blood vessels and increase a sense of calm. For nerves, try bath soaks containing geranium, vanilla, jasmine, peppermint, lavender and seaweed.

Aching muscles
Try a ten- to fifteen-minute warm bath (92°–102°) so muscles relax slowly. For muscle relaxation try bath products containing peppermint, primrose, lemon, bergamot, rosemary and cypress.

For exhaustion
Try a warm bath for ten to fifteen minutes. To ease into sleep try bath products with lavender, chamomile, rose and neroli (a classic scent in fragrances).

To energize
Soak in a bubble bath with citrus such as lemon, orange or grapefruit. Other botanicals to lift your spirits are peppermint, bergamot, patchouli, rosemary or eucalyptus.

TIP

Products that say "made for a woman" really mean made for a woman. A woman's perspiration has a higher pH level (more alkaline) than a man's. These products are designed to counteract this condition.

For a stiff back

Try a five- to ten- minute hot bath (102°–104° F). Dip a small towel in diluted soothing oils of menthol, eucalyptus, juniper, peppermint and lavender. Wrap it around your neck or place it behind your back.

Bathe your cold away

Coming down with a cold? Try this healing bath. Before you fill the tub add four tablespoons of dried lavender, two tablespoons of dried ginger powder, four tablespoons of dried rosemary and two tablespoons of dried eucalyptus leaves.

Here are some botanicals you may like and how they affect your body and mind:

Each botanical is an herb in essential-oil form. These essential oils are widely available in bath and body shops, health food stores, spa shops and even some supermarkets.

BASIL reduces nervous tension and relieves mental fatigue.

BAY acts as a decongestant and is good for a cold.

CALENDULA relieves inflammation and irritation.

CHAMOMILE calms the nervous system, soothes inflammation and relieves pain.

CLOVE stimulates and relieves muscle and nerve tension.

JUNIPER stimulates the nervous system and relieves fatigue.

LAVENDER calms. It relieves tension aches and muscle pains.

LEMON stimulates circulation and revives skin tone.

PEPPERMINT helps relieve headaches, fatigue, and tight muscles.

ROSE relieves headaches and improves circulation.

ROSEMARY tones the skin, stimulates circulation and relieves nervous tension and tight muscles.

SAGE relieves fatigue and nervous tension.

VETIVER relieves anxiety and nervous tension as well as muscle aches and pains.

YLANG YLANG calms nerves and relieves muscle knots and aches.

The power of aromatherapy

Smells not only affect us emotionally but physically. Actually, our sense of taste is made up of about 90% smell. When you use aromatherapy products on your body, you will enjoy the benefits all day. Here are a few smells that can give you a boost, calm you down or even make you think more clearly:

- To reduce anxiety, breathe in scents of green apple, cucumber, sandalwood or cedar.

TIPS

Limit your bath to a maximum of twenty minutes. Water that's too hot can dry your skin, irritate it and even rupture capillaries. The hotter the bath, the shorter the time you should spend in it.

Make your own bath oils by mixing ten to twelve drops of a concentrated, scented essential oil into a neutral oil such as almond or avocado. Then pour into your bath. If you are mixing scents and botanicals for healing, be sure to test a drop of each mixed together to see if the combination smells good. For the best aroma, it's best to mix just a few scents together.

After a bath, allow yourself ten minutes or so to lie down and relax. Make your transition back into the real world as gentle as possible.

- To increase alertness, inhale scents of peppermint or jasmine.
- To increase energy and stimulate, smell scents in peppermint, menthol, eucalyptus, lemon, vanilla, evergreen, fir, pine or spruce.
- For quiet focus, try lavender, frankincense, sandalwood, rose, cedar or myrrh.
- To help you go to sleep, smell scents in lavender or vanilla.
- To increase understanding of what you learn, smell scents of mixed florals.
- For concentration, breathe in rosemary, peppermint, basil, ginger or juniper.
- To decrease appetite, inhale scents of banana, green apple or peppermint.

Native Americans have burned herbs for centuries. Sage is burned to cleanse the mind, heart and home. Sweetgrass is burned to call good spirits. An easy way to burn these scents is with incense. Always buy quality incense—it smells much better.

Fragrance and performing

The more heated you become, the stronger your scent. If you wear a fragrance when performing, choose a subtle scent. Scent is released when fragrance heats up. So use it sparingly on pulse points—behind the knees, the crease of your elbow and on the wrist. Try a scented body lotion for a softer scent. If you are allergic to fragrance on your skin but love to have a scent, spray a little on your hairbrush and brush the scent into your hair. Another way is to spray the scent in the air in front of you and then walk into the scented mist. The aroma falls lightly onto your clothes and keeps you softly fresh all day. Store fragrance out of the sun and away from heat and moisture. Fragrance can be very refreshing to use when stored in the fridge.

The inspiration of color

It has been proven that color, like smell, has a strong effect on your mood. Make *color therapy* a part of your life. Drink a glass of red cranberry juice in the morning to get moving. Wear blue to relax when you feel stressed, or orange to help cheer you up. Add some green to help you focus, or stimulate your mind with a little yellow. You can use the power of color just by changing socks, tights and scarves, even your underwear. Use color for a good feeling and for fun.

Here are the ways that colors set a mood:
To inspire energy and boost confidence use *red*.
To stimulate the mind and feel inspired use *yellow*.
To relieve tension, feel calm and focused use *green*.

To cheer up, feel optimistic and increase enthusiasm use *orange*.

To clear your mind and increase creativity use violet or *purple*.

To unwind, relax and feel cool use *blue*.

Feel romantic and excited in *pink*.

Hair Care

How you care for your hair plays a big role in the health of your hair

Treat your scalp right

The condition of your scalp greatly affects the growth and health of your hair. Be sure to condition your scalp to strengthen hair and prevent dry scalp flakes. Before washing your hair, massage the scalp with the soft part of the fingertips to work out oil and dead skin. A great treatment the night before washing is to massage a few drops of olive or jojoba oil into your scalp, then brush through hair. This will treat both the hair and scalp.

The wash out

Keep your hair clean. Oil, dirt, dust, soap residue and styling products can make your hair look dull. Wash hair with shampoo that's right for your hair type. Massage shampoo into hair by squeezing it into the hair like you are squeezing a sponge. Work shampoo into hair and begin gently massaging scalp. Rinse and do not reapply unless hair is very oily. If dandruff is a problem, try a *conditioning* dandruff shampoo. They smell better and are gentler on your hair. Wash with water that's warm but not too hot, which can dry your scalp. The best time to wash your hair is at night. Pollutants and irritants collect in your hair through out the day and can be transferred to your pillow at night. This can cause red, puffy or watery eyes as well as skin rashes.

Condition it

Follow with a conditioner and use fingers to detangle before rinsing. Be sure to rinse out all of the conditioner. Breakouts and pimples on the back have been caused by not thoroughly rinsing out the conditioner. Dry hair can lack shine and break easily.

Drying out

Do not leave your hair wrapped in a towel for too long. It can dry hair to the point of damage and create a frizzy appearance when dry. Avoid rubbing your hair with a towel, which creates friction and roughs up the cuticle making hair look dull. Instead, gently squeeze out the water and pat hair with a towel. It is better to use a wide-tooth comb to further detangle wet hair.

Wet hair is very fragile and can break easily, especially when brushed. **Never brush wet hair!** Avoid pulling hair back tight when wet for the same reason. Washing and drying hair at night will help it look more sleek the next day and will get you off and running faster in the morning. An extra benefit to bathing at night is that it's a great way to help you fall sleep. When blow-drying, finish with your dryer on the cool setting for about two minutes to help smooth hair and add shine. Add body by drying your hair upside down the last two minutes of drying time. Be sure to use styling products at the roots of the hair, not on top. This prevents hair from becoming weighted down and provides lift at the scalp, adding volume.

The brush out

The right hairbrush can make a big difference in the health of your hair. Professional stylists say to change hairbrushes once a year. Old, out-of-shape bristles can break by scraping against the follicle at the scalp. Boar bristle brushes are great for the scalp, as they increase circulation and move oil through the hair. They also last longer than metal or plastic ones. Be sure to wash hairbrushes at least once a week—dirty brushes can quickly make your hair look dirty and dull. Use a comb to remove hair from the bristles, then wash the brush with shampoo or liquid soap, rinsing until clean. Always brush hair starting at the ends and work up to the scalp.

Growing out

Does your hair seem fuller and healthier in the summer? It may be because hair grows faster in warm weather. If you have been trying for long locks *forever*, remember that fine hair does not grow as fast as thick or coarse hair.

Don't stress your locks

When rehearsing, auditioning and performing, hair is often best kept off the face. Wearing hair pulled back tight in a ponytail or bun can put stress around the hairline and cause hair to break or fall out. Signs of this are a receding hairline or

Save Damaged Locks

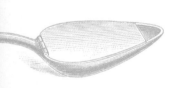

Try this quick natural conditioning treatment to save damaged locks

- In a blender, mix one avocado, one egg white and two tablespoons of olive oil. Blend thoroughly and apply to wet or dry hair. Put on a shower cap and sit in the sun for twenty minutes to warm. Wash out mixture with shampoo and warm water, then condition hair.

- To remove a styling product and shampoo build-up, try rinsing hair with one part vinegar or lemon juice to twenty parts water.

patches of short hairs around the face where breakage has occurred. To prevent this, try to mix up hairstyles. Use a large cloth scrunchie from time to time instead of a pony band and vary with hair clips. Claw and banana clasps have teeth that can become worn, shredding and tearing hair. File down rough edges on teeth to prevent breakage. Stress, vitamin deficiency and hormone changes can trigger hair loss as well. Hair naturally falls out in small amounts, but if you notice an increase in hair loss be sure to see a doctor. Each hair lives from two to six years and is then replaced by a new one. Average daily hair loss can be from twenty to one hundred hairs.

Feed your hair? New studies have shown that going more than four hours between meals without food can reduce the energy available to your hair follicles. It's starving your hair! . . . which can create weaker strands and uneven cuticles.

Hand & Nail Care

Hands are a very important part of beauty. We express thoughts and emotions with them. Our age, character and interests all show in our hands. Take pride in your hands and pamper them. The first impression people have of you is your face; the second, your hands.

At-home manicure

Once a week, soak hands in warm, natural oil such as olive or sesame. Wash them with lukewarm water and use a nailbrush with soap to remove dirt and grime under your nails (cleaning under your nails regularly is important to prevent the spread of germs). Scratch your nails over a soft bar of soap and wash in warm water if you don't have a brush. This also works well if you are gardening—to prevent dirt from getting under nails, don't wash away the soap. If you have stains on your nails, use a little lemon juice with hydrogen peroxide on your brush while scrubbing. After soaking, gently push back the cuticles with a wet washcloth. Do not cut cuticles, as they protect the nail from being damaged by bacteria, fungus, and irritating chemicals. File nails in one direction, instead of back and forth, to avoid weakening. File nails in a round or square shape, not pointed.

Nail polish can protect nails. Apply a natural soft beige or pink nail color for most performances. Theme nails can be worn to match specific costuming, but not if you have costume changes that will clash with the nail color. Be sure to use a base coat to protect the nail from staining. Touch up nails if the polish chips, instead of removing all nail color with polish remover. Nail polish remover can be drying and is best used only when a complete manicure is needed. Sun exposure can cause some polishes to turn yellow.

3
Makeup Basics for Natural Daylight Looks

In this chapter you will find the perfect makeup for natural light. Whether you need a soft no-makeup look, a professional application for an audition, pageant interview or outdoor performance, the following steps will insure you look your best naturally. Makeup for photographed headshots, a must for any professional performer, will also be included as this is a look that shows the real you—but at your very best.

Knowing your personal complimentary colors will keep you looking polished any time, even on the stage of life. Daylight can be unforgiving, requiring a light hand, perfect blending and foundation shades exactly matched to your skin's undertone.

Match foundation colors to your skin

One of the trickiest cosmetics to match to your skin is foundation. The match should be as close to perfection as possible. To match your skin, you must first understand what your skin undertone is. To find it, hold the underside of your wrist facing upward in good light.

- Do you have a golden, yellow, orange, olive, or bronze cast to your skin?
  If you do, your skin has a **warm undertone**.

- Do you have a pink, rosy/beige, or red/brown cast to your skin?
  If you do, your skin has a **cool undertone**.

If you are still confused, remember that 75% of us fall into the warm category. When it comes to choosing a foundation, concealer and powder, always choose shades with your same undertone. A great way to test foundation shades is to apply a swipe of foundation down your jawbone onto your neck (the neck gets very little sun and shows your true skin shade.) See if the shade blends well into the skin tone on your neck. This will help prevent your face from looking a different color from your body.

Note: If your face color is *much* darker than your neck, match your face color to your shoulder and chest. Blend the foundation evenly onto your neck. Allow the foundation to sit a minute, as many change color as they warm to the skin. Always check the match out in daylight or under a very bright lamp.

Correct with Color

Powder can be a great corrector to adjust skin color. Because of its sheer texture, it can look more natural than correcting with foundation. If your skin is very pink, dust a yellow-undertone powder over the foundation to tone down and correct redness. If foundation is too light, dust powder one shade darker over foundation to deepen.

Choosing Cosmetic Colors

With so many colors and shades of lipstick, shadow, and cheek colors available, making a decision on what looks best can be very confusing. Most makeup artists follow only one rule, *the warm/cool undertone theory.*

When it comes to choosing the right lip, cheek and eye colors it helps to remember that colors in your natural undertone will look best against your skin. However, you might feel washed-out in your natural undertone colors. Professional makeup artists will tell you that anyone can wear any color as long as you understand the effect that color has against your skin. The opposite undertone from your skin tone adds more drama and will look stronger and more intense.

Here are some guidelines for you to follow

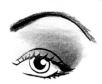 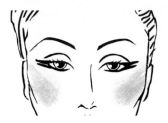 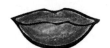

Eye shadows Cheek shades Lip shades

For a warm undertone NATURAL LOOK

black, charcoal brown	orange, corals, orange/brown	orange, corals, orange/brown
all golden or orange browns	peach, golden brown, bronze	peach, golden brown, bronze
peach, khaki, orange, yellow	red/orange, red/brown	red/orange, red/brown
green, gold, cream	gold, yellow/beige	gold, yellow/beige

For a warm undertone DRAMATIC LOOK

gray/black, plum/brown	pink, mauve, plum	all pinks, pink/brown, plum
purple, blue, lavender, mauve	purple/brown, pink/brown	purple/brown mauve, rose
pink, rose, silver, white	rose, burgundy	burgundy blue/red, silver/white

For a cool undertone NATURAL LOOK

gray/black, plum/brown	pink, mauve, plum	all pinks, pink/brown, plum
purple, blue, lavender, mauve	purple/brown, pink/brown	purple/brown, mauve, rose
pink, rose, silver, white	rose, burgundy	burgundy, blue red, silver/white

For a cool undertone DRAMATIC LOOK

black, charcoal brown	orange, corals, orange/brown	orange, corals, orange/brown
all golden or orange browns	peach, golden brown, bronze	peach, golden brown, bronze
peach, khaki, orange	red/orange, red/brown, gold	red/orange, red/brown, gold
yellow green, gold, cream	yellow/beige	yellow/beige

Choose shadow and eye liner colors that bring out your eye tones

BLUE EYES	**GREEN EYES**	**HAZEL EYES**	**BROWN EYES**
yellow/brown	red/brown	red/brown	red/brown
blue/gray	khaki, purple	true green	orange, bronze
gray/black, mauve	plum/brown	orange/peach	golden/brown
silver, white	lavender	purple	plum/brown
(khaki and wheat	peach, pink	rose, pink	black, gold
bring out the gray			
in blue eyes)			

Colors that bring out your hair tones:

Bring out highlights in your hair by using a shimmer powder highlighter on eyelids, under brows, and on cheekbones. For lips, add a shimmer lip gloss to highlight the center of your lips.

- If your hair has *golden* or *red highlights*, use a golden shimmer highlighter.
- If your hair has *platinum highlights*, use a white/silver shimmer highlighter.

To choose clothes that will blend with your makeup color, follow this easy system:

- *Warm* undertone makeup colors go best with clothing colors in red, blue, brown, khaki, orange, peach, gold, yellow, beige, cream, black or white.
- *Cool* makeup colors go best with clothing colors in purple, lavender, mauve, indigo (between blue and purple), pink, rose, silver gray, green, black or white.

TIPS

If you are wearing a red lipstick for the first time, try to find a red that's in your natural warm or cool undertone. The color, although bright, will look softer and you will get used to the look more easily. Very light lips look best in the dramatic-look undertones. Try to keep lips, cheeks and nail shades all in the same color family. Remember when it comes to foundations, concealers and powders, the choices are always in your natural skin undertone.

Notice how all makeup colors go with black and white? That's because these are non-colors on the color wheel, therefore work with all color undertones.

Cosmetic Products & What They Do

There are so many choices! Knowing the types and formulas of cosmetics and their intended use is very important to insure the best results.

To make shopping easier, use the following information to help you make the right choices. Remember, when it comes to performing, auditioning, interviewing or being photographed, **oil-free products work best**. When your skin perspires, excess oil is produced. To create a flawless canvas use oil-free products, starting with a moisturizer to prime the skin, then liquid foundation to even out the complexion and set with a translucent powder to help your makeup stay fresh and in place.

Foundations

Moisture tint—a sheer foundation that provides moisturizing benefits and minimal coverage. Best for normal to dry skin types.

Gel bronzer—a sheer tinted gel that provides a bronze or tan look. It provides no coverage but can disguise freckles and discoloration. It is usually is oil-free. Best for all skin types.

Mousse foundation—a whipped foundation with light to medium coverage. Most contain oil. Best for normal to dry skin types.

Cream foundation—a thick cream foundation that comes in a jar, tube, compact or stick (like a large lipstick container). Provides medium to full coverage. Most cream foundations contain oil, and can become shiny on stage. Best for normal to dry skin types.

Liquid foundation—formulas and amount of coverage varies in these foundations. They are the most common choice of foundation types and best to create a flawless natural look. Some contain a lot of oil and some are oil-free, so check the label to know the type of formula you're getting. For performing, use oil-free medium-to-full coverage liquid.

Compact powder makeup—also known as dual finish (foundation and powder in one), cake or pancake makeup. This foundation type can be used wet for light coverage or dry for heavy coverage. It is excellent for photography, but be careful as some do contain oil. Check the label. Dual finish makeup has a matte finish and works well for most skin types. Oily skin types should avoid daily use of this type; because of its thickness it can irritate pores and be difficult to touch up.

Foundation primer—a liquid in a sheer white shade. It is used under foundation to even out skin discoloration. Some primers help foundation stay on better. Many makeup artists use this product on rough, blotched, uneven or wrinkled skin.

TIP

Apply all foundations with clean fingers or a sponge, with gentle downward strokes. Since that's the direction your hair grows, you get smoother coverage. To thin out foundation, apply it using a moist sponge with a little water in it or moisturizer if skin is dry. Keep two shades of foundation, one for summer and one for your winter skin color and then mix as needed. Always apply foundation on top of moisturized skin. Dry skin can absorb foundation, which is why many people say that their foundation fades as the day goes on.

Concealers

Known as cover-ups, camouflage creams and concealers, these come in a stick, pot, wand or tube. These contain oil and should only be used to conceal under eye circles for normal to oily skin types. Yellowish shades look natural against most skin tones and are best for covering under-eye darkness. Some come in a mint/green color and are designed for covering ruddy or red skin blotches and purple under-eye darkness. Some come in pink/rose and are designed to add color to sallow, olive complexions. Some concealers come in oil-free formulas that are medicated to cover blemishes.

Powders

Loose powder—which comes in a large container, is designed for setting foundation. For stage, use oil-free powder to prevent shine breakthrough. Loose powder is usually translucent (sheer) and can be moisturizing for normal to dry skin types (a little oil in loose powder will create a dewy finish), or oil control/oil-free for normal to oily skin types (this has a matte finish). Apply entirely over foundation with a powder puff, sponge or large, thick, soft-hair powder brush. For smoother coverage, apply in downward strokes, the direction your hair grows. Avoid daily powdering under eyes which has a drying effect.

Compact powder—which comes pressed in cake form inside a compact, is designed for touch-ups. Best for on-the-go use and to powder breakthrough shine.

Lipsticks

Lipstick comes in sheer gloss, liquid, cream or matte formulas. Lipsticks that stain the lips and matte formulas are the longest lasting, but can be drying.

Cheek Color

Cheek color comes in a cake powder form that's matte or frosted. Matte formulas are best for a natural look. Rich pigments used in a matte formula are best for stage. Cake powder color is the most common choice and is for all skin types. Other choices include cream (for dry skin), gel (to stain cheeks) and loose powder (like a bronzer).

Eye Shadow

Cake/powder—which is the most common choice, works for all skin types. These come in matte (no shine), translucent (sheer), frost (shiny) and sparkly (with glitter). Remember, shadows rich in pigment (can be used wet or dry) are best for the stage.

TIPS

For precise application, concealers are best applied with a synthetic, small, flat brush or with a clean finger. To cover, gently pat concealer on the spot, blending out at the outer edges until invisible.

As in all your cosmetics, remember to keep sponges, brushes and puffs clean to avoid bacteria build-up.

Cream—which in most cases is used by dry skin types. Many creams are waterproof and most have a little shine. Best applied with a sponge applicator, but clean fingers are fine too. Cream eye shadow can be difficult to apply and blend when using more than one color. Soft shades look best. Cream is not advised for performing, because heat can cause creases.

Gel or liquids—which are sheer, provide only a tint to the lid. These are long lasting but can crease and are difficult to use when applying more than one color. Not for performing.

Easy Natural Makeup for Daylight

Here is an easy ten-minute face to keep your looks up and your stress down. It's perfect for those who want to look completely natural yet polished.

- Prepare your canvas: cleanse and moisturize, following the skin care steps described in chapter one.

- Apply a small dab of foundation just where you need to cover a few imperfections (around lips, nose, over eyelids and on dark spots).

- Pat then blend concealer on under-eye dark circles to create a fresh, rested look.

- Powder your face and eyelids, to create a smooth, long-lasting finish.

- If lips are narrow or small and need filling out, shaping or a more defined lip line, correct it with a lip pencil in the same color as your lips. Apply a sheer lipstick that has a little shimmer to add liveliness to the face. Light to medium sheer tones look best with a natural face. Brighten and add color to the face by using a sheer lipstick shade in the opposite color of your skin tone.

- Dust the apples of your cheeks with cheek color in the same undertone (warm or cool) as lips, and apply slightly above and across eye crease.

- Highlight with a sheer shimmer powder under brows, on eyelids, inner eye corners and cheekbones. It will brighten and whiten eyes as well as add radiance to the skin.

- Define brows (see page 60) to shape eyes and add balance to the face.

- Curl eyelashes with a lash curler and apply black mascara to draw attention to eyes. Those with fair skin and white toned blonde hair should use dark brown mascara.

TIPS

To find the apples of your cheeks, smile. The round balls of your cheeks are the apples. To avoid applying too much cheek color, after it's on the brush, shake off the excess on a tissue before applying to your cheeks.

For a more natural look, use shimmer powder in your skin undertone.

For perfectly curled lashes, try the *triple squeeze*. Place the open curler on the upper lashes near the roots and hold your lashes between the two rims. Squeeze gently for five seconds. Release the curler and move it to the center of the lashes and squeeze, then toward the outer part of the lash and squeeze again. The result? Beautiful curled lashes.

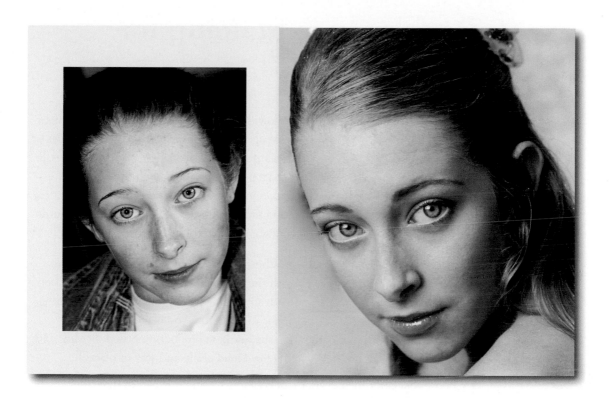

Good looks on the go

Being always on the go doesn't leave a lot of time for freshening up before rehearsal. Makeup combined with perspiration can cause skin problems, so here are a few tips for beautiful skin and great looks on the go.

Before you leave the house prepare your on-the-go tote bag. Inside your tote keep trial-size containers or fill up small bottles with face wash, toner and moisturizer. Also carry mints, aspirin, adhesive bandages, bobby pins, hair ties, hairspray, hairbrush, body lotion, safety pins, feminine needs, cotton swabs and cosmetic cotton pads. Place it all in your tote bag and include extra tights, bottled water and a healthy snack such as a health bar or almonds. (See page 85, chapter five, for a detailed list of tote bag necessities.)

Before rehearsal, class or practice, wash your face. First, wet a cosmetic cotton pad with water. Put a dime-sized amount of lotion face wash on the pad and rub it in a circular motion over your face to cleanse skin. Use a cotton pad with water to remove cleanser. Apply toner to cotton pad and stroke over the face to remove any residue and kill bacteria. Lastly, moisturize with an oil-free moisturizer. Remember perspiration produces more oil, so even dry skin might need to use an oil-free moisturizer when exercising. To keep up your good looks, leave color on the lips and eyes when cleansing. Those areas do not perspire.

TIP

Find travel size products at your local drug store or pick up some of your favorite skin care samples at department store cosmetic counters.

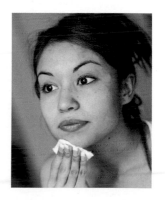

Performance Makeup for Natural Light

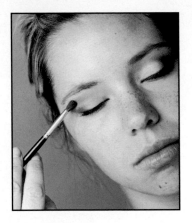

Follow these steps for perfect, polished daylight makeup. Perfect for drill, cheer, twirl, parades or pageant interviews. Daylight performances still need a polished makeup look. Remember the importance of a light hand and careful blending. After proper skin care (use a sunscreen if out in sunlight), follow these easy steps:

• When applying performance makeup, start with the eye makeup first. This makes it easier to clean up under-eye messes that occur during application. Before you begin, cover eyelid imperfections with foundation or a shadow base product if needed. Set lids with oil-free face powder to help eye shadow blend easily and stay in place.

• Choose your color theme—warm or cool tones—and stay within that color palette, not only for eyes, but cheeks and lips too. If you're performing and have many costume changes, use neutrals from the warm color tones. Decide first which lipstick color you plan to wear, and build the color theme around that shade.

• Begin with the darkest shadow shade. Try a dark brown (in the warm/neutral palette) or plum/brown (in the cool palette). Apply at the outer corner of the eye, stopping slightly above crease. Then blend half way in toward nose to contour.

• Brush on a medium tone in soft peachy/brown (warm/neutral) or rosy/brown (cool) across eye bone (the top of the eye socket) just above the crease of the lid, blending in edges of dark shadow. This lifts eyes.

• Highlight across inner half of lid and under eyebrow, a soft shiny cream tone (warm/neutral) or white/pink (cool) shadow.

• Line the eyes with dark shadow, used wet with a pointy brush, or use a liquid liner. Create soft thin lines. For an even softer look, try a black cake liner half way across the top of your lid, sweeping slightly up at the outer side towards the eye crease, and a brown cake liner under outer half of the bottom lashes. Don't continue the line into the corners where the upper and lower liners meet, so eyes look wider. Never line the ridge of the lower lid above lower lash roots. The eyes will look small and closed. A white pencil applied on the ridge above the lower lash roots can brighten, whiten and open eyes.

TIPS

To keep eye shadow from falling and smudging under the eyes, tap the brush on a tissue to remove excess color before applying.

In sunlight, use less liner. To prevent running, use an eye-liner sealer. This is a clear liquid, used in place of water, on a liner brush with eye shadow or cake liner. This seals the liner so it's water resistant. (See my website, modedion.com, for this product.) Stay away from pencil liners as most contain oil that melts easily under heat.

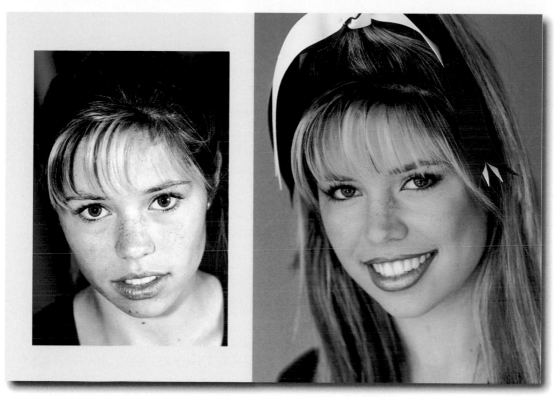

The look of cool tones

- Shape brows with cake or pencil brow liner. For brunettes, use the same color as your hair and for blondes use one shade darker. (See the section in chapter four titled "Brows frame your eyes.")

- Clean up any fallen shadow under eyes with eye makeup remover on a Q-tip®.

- Apply oil-free foundation over areas that you feel need coverage. Most faces need foundation along the sides of the nose, cheeks, chin (to cover redness), eyelids, lips and over spots and blemishes. Use a foundation shade that is an exact match to your skin color. Blend a little onto your throat for even color.

- Apply concealer over under-eye darkness only where needed.

- Use a loose oil-free face powder. To control shine longer, use a cosmetic cotton pad or powder puff to apply powder. Press in all over the face. Avoid the eye area, where dryness can occur as the day goes on. Finish by buffing off excess powder over face with a large powder makeup brush.

- Apply black mascara, starting with bottom lashes. Wiggle the wand back and forth at the roots to distribute mascara evenly and separate lashes. Put on three coats. If you are wearing false lashes, put on only one coat.

- Contour cheeks with soft pink/brown cheek color. Start at the center of your ear blending toward the base of your nostril. Stop two fingers away from the

TIPS

In natural light, it is best *not* to blend a layer of foundation all over the face. It can look too heavy and unnatural.

By pressing on powder, you seal foundation, prevent running and control shine from perspiration under hot sunlight. Always have a powder compact or blotting papers in your tote for quick touch-ups.

nose in a sweep up around the apples of your cheeks. Blend color into the temples, the sides of forehead, lightly on center of the chin and along the sides of the nose. This defines the face and adds color to the skin.

TIP

Apply lip liner with short slow strokes looking one stroke ahead as you line. Keep a rounded lip at the top and close lips together to line at mouth corners. Smile to see if corners meet. Be sure lips are full at the sides.

- Add life to the cheeks by smiling to define apples of cheeks, and apply a matte, sheer, natural-looking cheek color in peach (warm), sheer red (neutral) or pink (cool) shade. To avoid applying too much cheek color, apply it at the end of your makeup application. Applying it last helps you control the amount of color really needed on the cheeks.

- Line lips in a natural tone of peach/brown (warm), red/brown (neutral), or pink/brown (cool) lip pencil. Fill in entire lip with lip pencil to increase lipstick staying power.

- With a lip brush, apply lipstick all over lips. Use a bright *sheer* color in coral/peach (warm), clear red (neutral) or pink/rose (cool). Sheer shades look glossier and natural.

- Optional: add a little shimmer to create the look of natural radiance. Apply a sparkly, shiny gloss just to center of upper and lower lip. Add a shimmer powder to upper cheekbones, at center of lid and under eyebrow arch. Exposed skin on the chest, shoulders, back or stomach can look smooth and radiant when shiny sheer powder is lightly applied to catch sunlight.

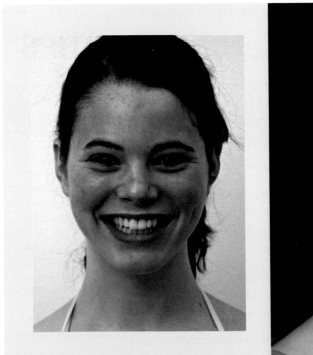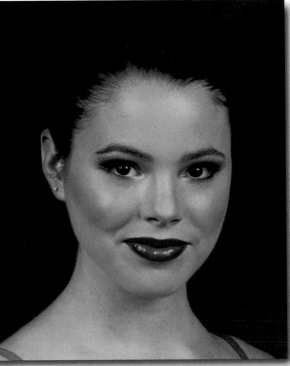

The look of warm tones

Daylight Pageant Makeup

The pageant interview is a time to focus away from the way you *look* and more on *you*. That means keeping your makeup polished and professional (not overdone) so that it does not distract the interviewer. Follow the rules above but keep the look a bit more natural. Use a soft color on the lips. Shape and define lips with a natural lip liner and fill in with soft lip color in pink or peach. Mixing the two together makes a versatile color that looks great on everyone. I like to mix shimmer pink lipstick or gloss with a beige/peach clear gloss on top. These colors look beautiful together and on all skin tones, really adding life to the face. For more information, see chapter five.

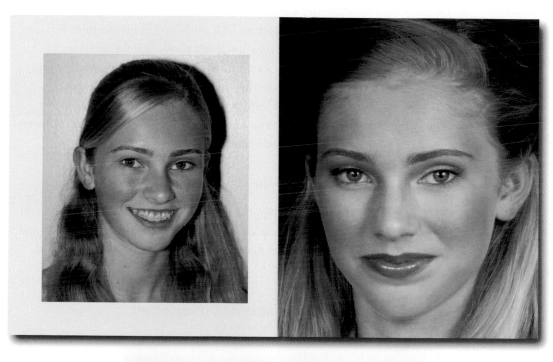

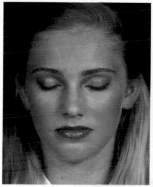
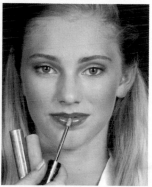

Audition Makeup

Makeup is a part of performing. Performers are expected to know how to apply their own makeup. Knowing and following industry expectations distinguishes the amateurs from the professionals.

Auditioning for videos, commercials and industrials

When you are putting on makeup for an audition, the most important thing to remember is the kind of job you are auditioning for and making sure your look is appropriate for that job.

Your appearance can play a big part in the judge's decision. Are you auditioning for a teen pop star, rapper or a glamorous diva? Teen pop stars look for young and fresh looks so makeup needs to look softer and more youthful. Hip hop or rap is a street look with stronger eyes and softer glossy lips; for glamour, do rich lips and defined eyes. Keep the look you want to achieve in mind. Performers are most likely to be videotaped when they have made the last cut. Appearing in the right makeup for the job and learning to skillfully apply your makeup in complimentary colors, shows you're a professional. Watch music videos and dancers in commercials—and observe the style and makeup they wear.

Auditions for a dance company

The sort of dance and the personality of the company always direct the mood and look of dance company makeup. There are a few basic rules to follow for professional audition makeup. (Remember, if you make it to the final round, there is a good chance that you will be videotaped.)

Camera-ready makeup for videotaped auditions

Whether it's the videotaping of a performance or the taping of the final cut of an audition, these techniques will make sure you are camera ready. A good starting point is to follow the steps outlined in *Performance Makeup for Natural Light* (page 40). A few exceptions apply.

Eyes
Blend eye shadow colors in seamlessly. Go light on eyeliner and avoid black liner unless you want a more dramatic look. In most cases it's best to stay with soft colors like brown or gray. Do not let eyeliner meet at the inner and outer corners. Avoid lining the ridge above lower lash roots. Instead, use white pencil there to open and whiten eyes. A short row of false lashes can be used but keep the look natural.

Brows

Brows should be shaped and defined in a shade close to hair color. Avoid red/brown or orange/brown tones unless hair color is red.

Foundation

Unlike the perfect foundation facial match needed for daylight, video lights can make your face look lighter and washed out. Be sure to match foundation to shoulders and chest. Avoid foundations labeled "light reflective." These make your face look white under lights.

Concealer

Poor video lighting can create shadows beneath the eyes. Be sure under-eye dark circles are covered. Be careful that your concealer is not too light, as it tends to look white under eyes.

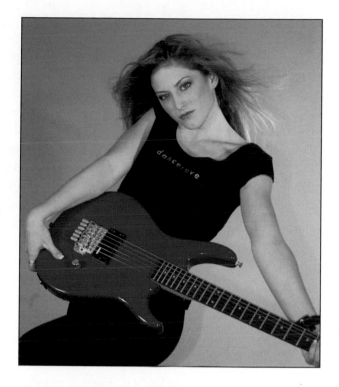

Powder

Choose a golden-toned translucent face powder, *slightly* darker than your face tone to add *just a bit* of color. Always keep a powder compact on hand for quick touch-ups.

Cheeks

Use enough matte cheek color to avoid looking pale and unhealthy. Make sure to use a little matte contour cheek color under cheekbones and along sides of nose (unless nose is long and narrow) to define features. On camera, a face can look more round and features can appear washed out.

Lips

Blend a cream formula lipstick into the lip pencil, so the color is seamless. For a softer line, apply pencil after lipstick. Blend liner into lipstick. Avoid pencils and lipsticks in true browns or plums—they can look muddy and bland on camera. Don't be afraid to play with color! Layering color can add life to the lips. Try pink lipstick with a peach gloss or sheer red with a beige/gold gloss.

False lashes

Use them if you need them. Smaller eyes and deeper skin tones can benefit from a row of natural-looking false lashes. Cut lashes in half for a more natural look.

Reflection

Beware of shiny jewelry and too much lip gloss. These reflect light, taking attention away from your performance.

TIP

Avoid shiny jewelry, glitter, sparkles, very glossy lips and shimmer on your face, as the camera picks up all reflection. (Music videos carefully light these extras so they don't catch too much reflection and overpower the look.)

Makeup for Men & Boys

Most men wear little if any makeup to auditions. Cover blemishes and other imperfections with a little foundation and set with powder. Even out brows, if needed, and hydrate lips with a lip balm. This is likely enough for any audition. On small stages used for dance competitions, however, men (teens and older) can use a bit more makeup. Conceal dark under-eye circles, cover blemishes or red, uneven skin using foundation *sparingly*, and set with face powder to control oily facial shine. Keep brows, as well as any other facial hair, well groomed and filled in lightly if needed. A light coating of mascara in dark brown can help draw attention to eyes. If lips are small or the lip line is uneven, use a natural flesh toned lip pencil to correct and a lip tint or lip balm to enhance lip color. The goal is, of course, to look as if there is no makeup.

Boys can conceal dark under-eye circles, shape brows and set face with powder. The most natural look is what's expected. (See chapter five, page 90, for more directions.)

Practice makes perfect

Auditioning can be a stressful experience. As with anything, the best way to reduce anxiety is preparation and practice. Try new colors and techniques when you're not under pressure and have time to experiment. Ask the opinion of others. Watch yourself on video and see how different colors look against your skin on camera.

Going Pro? It's Time for Professional Photos

The look, the prep and what to expect

You will be expected to have a headshot when auditioning for a professional job. This photograph should show you looking your very best in a natural makeup that enhances your good looks. If you sign with an agent or manager, either one will direct you to a photographer for pictures. If this is your first time and you would like to have pictures to send out for representation or work, here is a safe way to get started.

Find the right photographer

It's a good idea to interview the photographer and be sure you are comfortable with his style of work, even if it is one your agent has sent you to. In most cases headshots should be shot in black and white.

Sometimes a composite picture, a card with pictures of several looks such as casual, dance and dramatic, is requested. These photographs are shot in both black and white and color photography.

Many photographers have a favorite makeup artist they can recommend to assist you on the day of your photo shoot. When preparing for headshot photos, it's important to try a few different tops and looks so you have more to choose from. Be sure to experiment a bit. Often an idea that was just for fun turns out to be the unexpected best look of the day. It is usually best to stay away from a top with prints that distract from your face. Remember to bring only age- and job-appropriate clothing. If you are represented by an agent, ask what look he or she would like you to have.

The night before your photo shoot

Be sure all your clothes are clean, ironed and look great on you. Try on everything in front of the mirror. Move around and see how your shoulders, face and expressions work.

Be sure to pamper your skin the night before. Clean your face properly and use a gentle facial scrub so skin is smooth; then moisturize. Check the skin on your body, making sure you look smooth and healthy as well as free from any tan lines. Hair should be clean and trimmed for easy styling. Nails need to be clean and manicured in light-to-nude polish. Men should shave the night before to avoid redness, unless beard is *very heavy*. The most important beauty treatment you can get is a good night's sleep.

Pack a model's tote

A bag for emergencies is extremely important on a photo shoot. Be sure to pack the following: jewelry, shoes, several colors of tights, a small towel, a light robe, deodorant, tissues, a razor with a new blade, scissors, body lotion, tooth brush, Band Aids®, aspirin, a nail file, hairspray, hair brush and comb, water bottle, snack, small mirror, needle and thread, scotch tape (for hems) and your own makeup, including mascara and face powder (even if you have your own makeup artist). Be sure you have a map to the photo shoot and your appointment book with the pertinent phone numbers.

Plan to be a half hour early just in case you get lost or caught in traffic. Lateness is for amateurs; you are a professional.

The right makeup for the right look

Whether you have a makeup artist or plan to do your own, knowing the right colors and application for photography will keep you looking your best.

Here are a few guidelines to add for a polished, photo-ready face:

- Define, arch, and extend brows to look natural.

- Blend eye shadow in brown and peach tones. Line eyes lightly, especially under lower lashes, where too much liner can look overdone. Use a white eye pencil just above lower lash lid to open eyes.

- Add a very light dusting of shimmer powder at the inner eye corner, center of lid and brow arch. This really opens eyes.

- Mascara should be natural and brushed to look like real lashes. False lashes can be used as long as they are a natural length and thickness. To create more of a natural look, cut off a fourth of the false lash and apply the small cutting at the outer eye corner, which helps "lift" the eyes and still looks fresh. Always finish with mascara to weave your natural lashes into the false ones. Check for clumps.

- Keep foundation in golden tones and use concealer to cover under-eye dark circles and below nostrils to lift away shadows. Cover any uneven skin tones or flaws. This is one of the few special occasions when concealer can be used on the face as a cover-up. Powder well to set makeup and avoid shine.

- Use a pink/beige lip liner for a natural lip look, then brush on lipstick in a medium color tone. Lip lines should be undetectable. Gloss looks great and adds fullness, as do lipsticks with shimmer that highlight just the center of the lower and upper lip. Be sure to blend well.

- Flush cheeks and temples in a matte pink/peach neutral shade and lightly onto chin. Define features with a contour cheek color shade in pink/brown, at sides of nose, the cheekbones and jaw line. Blend well.

- Hair should be styled away from your face. Watch for loose strands and hair that distracts from your face.

Men's and boys' head shots

A natural look is very important. Focus on a well groomed, not a made-up, look. Shape and define brows. Even out skin and get rid of under-eye darkness with concealer, then set with face powder. Define features lightly with face contour cheek color shade.

Working with a photographer and posing

Let the photographer direct you. Ask what he or she would like you to do. Ninety-five percent of your look is expression! Lower your eyes, feel the mood, then slowly look up into the camera with energy. (If the light is too strong, look down and then up quickly with expression.)

Watch for a wrinkled forehead, showing too many teeth (move your lower jaw forward a bit to avoid this), too much gum, a chin too low (which makes a double chin and shadows under eyes) or a chin too high (the nostrils become pronounced). Be aware of eyes that are too big (a dead fish look) or squinted and lips that are too puckered (trying to be sexy). If you put your hands against the face, be careful not to push or wrinkle skin. Remember posture—chest up, shoulders down—breathe and relax.

Studio etiquette

Many photographers use a large piece of paper, called a backdrop, which hangs behind you on the wall. Wait for directions on where to stand on the paper before walking on it, as footprints and tears will ruin it. Lights and umbrellas may surround you. The photographer or assistant will do a light test by your face with a meter. During these tests you will hear a popping sound. This is to make sure the lights are perfect for a beautiful photo.

Ageless Beauty

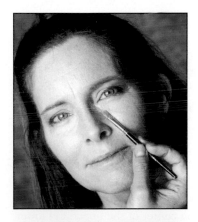

Daylight against mature skin can reveal brown spots, wrinkles and other skin flaws that only add years. Minor corrections, along with a few beauty tips, can truly enhance and add radiance.

Skin care

As stated in chapter one, the condition of your skin greatly depends on daily care. Hydrate face, including eyes, day and night. Never leave the house without sunscreen on your face.

Brow lift

Shaping the brows and lifting the ends slightly up and out will provide lift to the eyes.

Eye lift

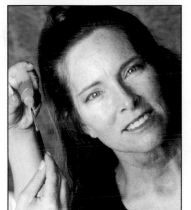

Define eyes with matte brown or plum eye shadow. Be sure to apply the dark shade at the outer corner stopping just above the crease. Balance eyes across eye bone just above crease with a matte natural beige shadow. Highlight with a matte soft pink/cream shadow onto

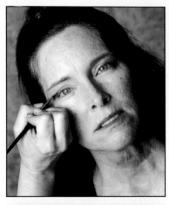

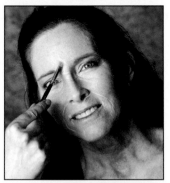

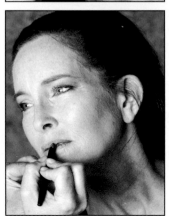

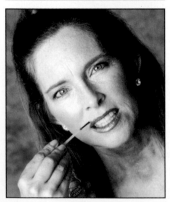

inner half of lid and under eyebrow. Blending is very important. Line eyes using the dark shade of the eye shadow on the upper lid. At the outer corner, point the line straight up toward the end of the brow. Avoid liner under lower lashes. If you must use liner there, be sure it is the beige shadow color applied wet. Clean up under eyes with a Q-tip® and apply eye cream to soften wrinkles.

White out

A white pencil is the perfect line filler. Draw a line through all wrinkles and into shadows at inner and outer corners of the eyes. Don't forget under the nostrils and the corners of lips to create lift. Blend in until untraceable with a small synthetic brush.

Foundation

Use a mineral cream makeup or liquid oil-free makeup in the correct skin tone. For ruddy complexions, use a golden undertone foundation to correct. Apply only where needed. Most faces need coverage at the sides of the forehead, sides of the nose, under nose and around lips and jawbone to cover imperfections from sun damage. Conceal only where needed especially at inner eye corner where shadows create darkness.

Radiance

Radiance is the key to youth. Apply a liquid or cream shimmer on cheekbones, apples of cheeks and center of forehead. Be sure it is sheer. A golden pink shimmer looks natural on most skintones.

Full lips

Full lips are a sign of youth. Fill out sides of mouth and round out lips for maximum fullness using lip pencil in a natural pink/beige shade. Fill in lips so the pencil is untraceable. Use a sheer lipstick that is glossy, two shades brighter than your own lips. Top the center of the upper and lower lip with a shimmer lipstick gloss. To avoid having lipstick run into lines around the mouth, seal with lipstick sealer (see *modedion.com*).

To set makeup

Use face powder lightly, just on the front (not the sides) of the face. Moisturizing powders or mineral powders create a more dewy finish.

Blush

Apply a light cheek color like pink or peach. Apply high on the apples of the cheeks, another sign of youth.

To look dewy and fresh

Add moisture with a face spray for a radiant finish.

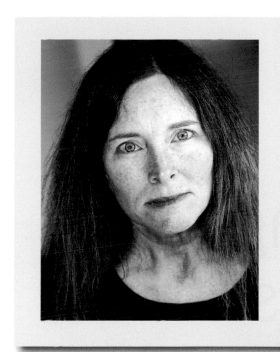

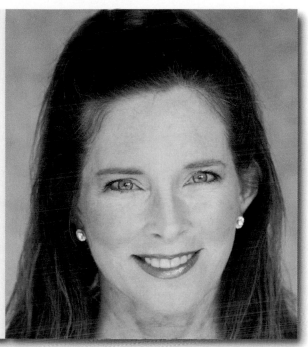

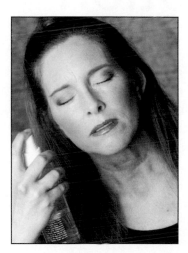

TIPS

For more of a glow, mix a little shimmer into your foundation.

Make your own face spray by mixing water and essential oil of rose, or just add rosehips from your garden. Add liquid minerals (gold, copper or silver) to help rejuvenate skin and improve circulation.

4
Sculpting Features to Perfection

N obody is perfect—not even the models and celebrities you see in magazines. The makeup artist's job is to create the illusion of perfection, and very few of us see the corrections that were made behind the scenes.

Makeup artistry is meant to enhance your natural features and invisibly correct any imperfections. When elements discussed in this chapter come together to correct and define the structure of the face, we call it "face physics." With these easy steps, as well as understanding how contouring and highlighting works, you can create the look of perfection just as the pros do.

You might ask why I am bringing up sculpting features now and not before the previous chapter, *Makeup Basics for Natural Daylight Looks*. In daylight, makeup should only enhance your natural beauty, and efforts to sculpt features could make you look overly made up. Evening and stage looks are under artificial light, which can wash out features and facial color. However, if you feel the need to sculpt features and make corrections to your daylight makeup look, when auditioning, performing or having your picture taken in color, use these techniques but with a lighter application.

Face Physics:
Correcting & Shaping Features

Here are the basic rules:

- Contouring with darker matte colors brings the focus in, and highlighting with bright, shimmery or light colors takes the focus out.

- Shape and define with contouring; lift and enhance with highlighting. Once you know this formula, application becomes much easier.

- The key is blending!

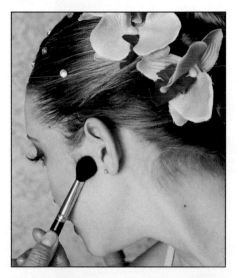

All facial shapes can use "face physics"—that is, they can benefit from contouring and highlighting. Contour features with a brown-toned cheek shade two or three shades deeper than your cheek color. I recommend a brown/pink cheek color for all skin tones except the deepest. Deep skin tones including mocha to espresso shades can benefit from a burgundy/brown cheek color for contouring. To apply contour color with precision, use a small check color brush or a large eye color brush. Some makeup artists contour facial features using a liquid foundation two or three shades darker than the natural foundation shade, and apply it using fingers or a large synthetic foundation brush. This method requires great care in blending so it looks natural. Highlight features by using a light matte face powder or a light shimmer liquid or powder with a medium fluffy brush.

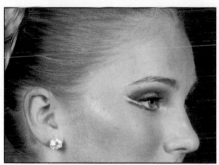

Create a defined cheekbone

Start at the center of your ear and blend down toward the base of your nostrils. Stop contouring about two fingers away from the nose (place two fingers straight up next to nose). Be sure to finish with an up-swing like a hook around the apple of your cheek. Keep in mind where the base of your cheekbone is as you blend down. To further lift the cheekbone, highlight the highest point. Start high at the outer temple and blend shimmer down the front of the face. Stop three fingers away from the side of your nose. Don't highlight the areas where you are prone to natural shine.

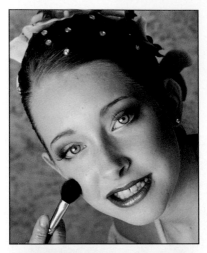

Flush cheek apples

Choose a bright cheek color in the same color family as lip color. Smile and apply to the apple (round part of the cheek), finishing slightly up on the cheekbone in a teardrop shape. Be very careful not to go up the cheekbone all the way as this will create a horizontal stripe of color.

Define the nose

To define the nose, lightly blend your contour shade from where the brow begins at the bridge of the nose down the sides of the nose to the tip. To bring out the bridge of the nose, use a light matte powder down the center of the nose line. A defined nose line can be very important when you are on a large stage where spotlights can wash away your features.

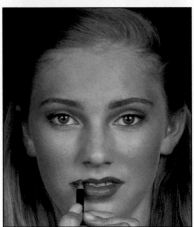

Fuller lips

Apply lip pencil one shade darker and slightly browner than lipstick color over whole lip. For example, with pink lipstick, use a pinky/brown pencil; with red lipstick, a red/brown pencil. The darker-tone pencil makes the outer lip line disappear and pulls lips down at the sides. But when the brighter lipstick shade is applied on top, the lips pull forward, creating a fuller looking lip. To create more fullness, the lip pencil may be left off the inner portion of the lips. Make sure the sides of the lips appear full in profile. Use the pencil to bring out the sides of the mouth where needed. To create even more fullness, highlight the center of the upper and lower lip with a light shimmer gloss or lipstick.

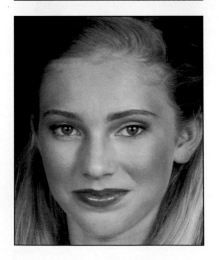

Contour a wide face

Follow the techniques for contouring cheekbones, then contour along the jawbone and up along the side of your hairline onto sides of the forehead. Apply blush in the brighter cheek color on apples of cheeks, but avoid applying this shade too high on the apple. Follow the full lip technique and shape lips wide and full at the sides to create a larger looking mouth. Keep the top bow of lips rounded, not pointy. If face is very round, arch lips to a slight point but keep the fullness of the mouth. Extend the brow line out at the end for more length, never rounded or swooping down. This helps provide balance to the face.

Highlight a long face

Use a shimmer face powder or pearly liquid on key spots to enhance cheekbones, under brows blending out to temples. Use a lighter shade matte face powder or foundation on chin and sides of forehead to widen face. Keep lip line round with a full width and curve.

For a high or pronounced forehead

Shade across the top of the forehead from your left temple to your right. Be sure to use a face powder or blot the area to reduce shine, as any shine or light reflection can further enhance the forehead.

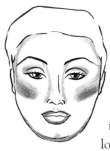

Conceal a double chin

Contour the area you want reduced by using a foundation one or two shades darker than that used for your face. After you apply the facial foundation in your skin color, pat and blend the darker foundation on top of the double chin and into the jaw line and onto the throat, so that it looks natural.

Cover scars, bruises and blemishes

Try using a medium to full coverage foundation before trying a heavy concealer formula. Concealers are thick, can look unnatural on the skin and may cause blemishes. If you are prone to breakouts, try a medicated blemish treatment concealer. Using a pointed-tipped makeup brush or your fingertip, pat a small amount of foundation on top of imperfection. Pat to cover, then blend the sides out into the skin until the edges are invisible. If the imperfection is still evident, pat a small amount of concealer on top of the area where more coverage is needed. Set with powder.

Cover dark under-eye circles

Finish applying all eye makeup and foundation. It is very important to be working on clean under-eye skin. Any residue from mascara or eye shadow flecks can melt as time progresses and further darken the under-eye area. Spread a light covering of foundation under the eye. For concealing, the best tool to use is a small synthetic brush. Fingers and sponges can be too wide to get into the key coverage area and can rub the makeup off the area you want to cover. Apply a very small amount of concealer, one shade lighter than the foundation, to the tip of the brush. The concealer should be a yellow tone so under-eye darkness won't look gray. Spread concealer only on the dark area, making sure edges blend into the foundation. Do not apply on the smile lines at the outer edges of your eyes to avoid a creased look. No heavy lining under the bottom lashes—try a brown liner beneath lower lashes instead of black, and line only half way to nose. Set liner with eyeliner sealer to prevent running.

Note: sometimes the under-eye area looks dark because of the shadow cast by puffiness. In this case, apply the concealer only under the area of the puff where the shadow is at the base.

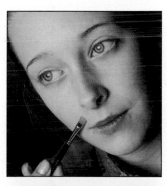

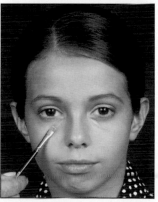

Eye Corrections

Do	**Don't**

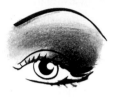

Apply neutral
colors that go with
everything.

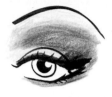

Don't apply more than three
shades at a time! No green or blue
shadow unless it is part of a theme.

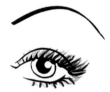

Comb out lashes.
Keep corners of eye open!

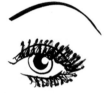

Don't use too much
mascara.

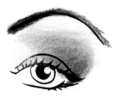

Use highlighter and glitter
in key light catching areas.

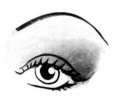

Don't apply too much highlighter
on lid, it makes you look puffy!

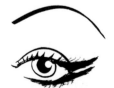

Keep corners of
eye open!

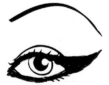

Don't use eyeliner all
around the eys.

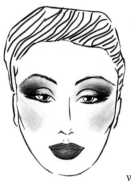

Close-set eyes

For eyes that are less than one eye length apart, eye shadow placement and brow shaping will make the difference. Be sure to highlight the inner half of eyelid and eye corner with white pencil or a light shimmer shadow. Apply the darkest eye shadow contour color at the outer corner, about one-fourth of the way onto eyelid, sweeping up and out just above crease. A medium shadow shade, applied slightly above the eye crease, should be blended only half way across the brow bone, sweeping up towards the end of the brow to pull the eyes outward. Highlight under brow from the arch out to the end. To help add space between eyes, brows should begin a bit further out from where eyes begin; some tweezing might be needed.

Highlighting corrects deep-set eyes

Find the dark areas of the eye and highlight, including the inner corner next to the nose. Never use a dark contour shadow in a crease or dark area of the eye. Remember: dark shades bring in and light shades bring out.

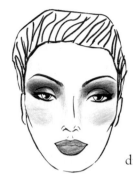

Wide-set eyes

For eyes that are more than one eye length apart, again, shadow and brow shaping will make the difference. To bring eyes closer, apply darkest eye shadow contour color along lash line, blending up into the crease, keeping away from inner corner of the lid. Apply a medium shade above crease and across to the inner half of the eye by the sides of the nose. Highlight under brow and onto inner lid. Extend brows further inward than where inner corner of eyes end.

Contouring corrects large eyelids

Reduce lid by starting at the outer edge of the eye. Apply a dark shadow across almost the entire eyelid leaving only the most inner part of the lid light. Blend the middle shadow shade slightly above eye crease across and into inner eye corner. Line across the entire lid. Highlight under brow and down the center of lid only.

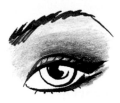

Small eyes

Liner makes the difference. To line, start at the end of the upper lashes sweeping out and up toward end of brow, stopping just above the crease. Line under bottom lashes starting at the center of your eye with a thin line and finish slightly beyond the end of the lash line. To create a longer, more opened eye, do not let lines meet at the outer corners. Use a white pencil to highlight the ridge of the lower lid and between the liners at the outer eye corner.

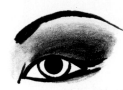

Eyes without a noticeable lid

These eyes are hooded or almond shaped (usually Asian eyes). First, blend a dark matte shadow three-quarters of the way across the eye just above crease. Then brush a medium shadow shade just above the dark shadow on the eye bone, blending in the edges. Lightest shadow is applied across entire lid and way up under the brow. For more definition apply black matte shadow at the outer-most corner blending to just above crease to lift. Line eyes with the same technique described on this page for *small eyes*. To draw attention to the lid and lift eyes apply a shimmer powder on center of lid near lashes and brow arch.

Nose Corrections

Contour a wide nose

First determine where the widest points are. Contour along nose, blending a thin line along the sides at the widest point. Blend contour color out into skin so the edges are invisible. A light beige eye shadow color or powder can work as well as the contour cheek color to shade sides.

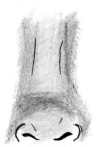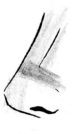

For a long nose

Use the same tools described for shaping a wide nose. Blend a line across the nose at the center, then blend out the sides of the line. This cuts the nose in half and creates a break in the long nose line. To shorten further, apply a little contour color to the very tip of the nose down to the base of the nostrils. You can create the look of a wider nose at narrow points by using a light matte face powder on the narrow parts of the nose. This reflects light and makes the area look larger.

Get rid of a bump in the center of the nose

Use the contour technique (above) but only contour across the bump.

Lip Corrections

Make small lips look larger

Trace around the edge of your natural lip line with a pencil in a shade darker than your lips. Fill in most of the lip with the pencil, which will prevent an unnatural-looking outer line. Turn your head to the side and be sure that the sides of your lips look full. With a lip brush apply a bright or shiny lipstick, reflecting light and making lips look fuller. Add a lip gloss or sparkling highlighter lipstick (like white, silver or gold) just in the center of the upper and lower lip. This reflects light out of the center and creates an even, fuller looking lip.

Reduce large lips

Around the inner lip, line your lips using a lip pencil two shades darker than your natural lip color. Apply a matte or deep color lipstick with a lip brush, blending with the lip pencil.

Correct crooked lips

Create balance with lip liner to match sides evenly.

If lips are too wide

Use concealer to cover corners where the lips end. Then line lips slightly inside the outer edge of the natural lip line at corners. Keep mouth closed when lining so you can easily see where the corners should end.

Lip lining and highlighting

When using lip liner, cover lips with foundation to create an even canvas. Use a lip pencil to line lips evenly, blending liner onto the lip so unattractive skinny outer lines won't show when lipstick wears off. Matching your lip pencil to a lipstick color can create a one-dimensional look. Use a lip pencil one shade darker and a bit more brown than your lipstick color, especially for reds, to tone down brightness and create the appearance of fuller lips.

To create fuller, more luscious lips, apply a lip gloss or shiny lipstick highlighter on the center of upper and lower lips.

Brows Frame Your Eyes

Before you paint your masterpiece, prepare a frame that sets off your beautiful expressive eyes. Start with tweezing the brows.

Have the right tools and know the rules:

- Pointy-tipped tweezers are the best to pull those stubborn little brow hairs.

- Before you begin, sterilize the tip of your tweezers with rubbing alcohol. Next sterilize the area you will be tweezing with astringent. This not only removes bacteria, but also removes oils from the skin that make tweezing hairs difficult.

- Pull hairs in the direction the hair grows. When hair is tweezed against hair growth the roots remain and look like little black dots.

- Avoid too much tweezing! Be especially careful when tweezing above the brow.

- For best results, draw the desired brow shape first, then brush brow hairs into the desired shape. Some artists use a white pencil to draw over areas they want to tweeze. The hairs disappear, making it easier to see what the brows will look like when hair is removed. This technique helps you to balance your eyebrows, making sure they will look even.

- Use a good magnifying mirror, and maintain brows with regular grooming.

How to shape brows

To understand how a brow should be shaped to best flatter your eyes and your face, it is important to know the standard brow-shaping formula:

Where your brow should begin: Place pencil alongside your nose pointing up and stopping at the inner corner of your eye. Your brows should begin here. To make your eyes look more open, tweeze the hairs that grow outside this area.

Where your brow should arch: Looking straight ahead, place pencil parallel to the center of eye pupil, pointing up. The arch should begin here. Tweeze out the hairs that are not a part of the brow line at this arch. This lifts and opens the eyes.

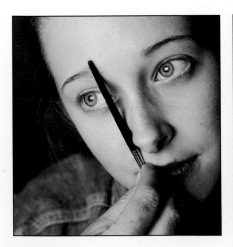

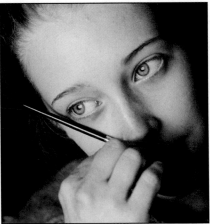

Where your brow should end: Place the pencil along side the nose, line to the outer corner of your eye and stop at the end of your brow. This is where your brow should end. Most people have brows that are too short, which makes the eyes look smaller. Be sure to extend brows to where they should end and avoid rounding down which can cause eyes to look droopy.

Treating unruly brows

Curly or wild brows need control. Apply a brow gel, hair gel or hair spray to a toothbrush or brow brush and brush where needed. Brows that are too long can be carefully trimmed with manicure scissors or other small scissors.

Droopy brows need to be brushed up and out. Try to clear away stray hairs that cause the droop.

Straight brows need to be tweezed at a slant, then rounded at the inner eye corner. Create a clean center with a high arch. Pencil in where needed.

Short brows need length—make sure brows begin and end as described above.

Full brows need to be brushed straight up and then tweezed as described above. Using a brow pencil, draw brows in the desired shape first before tweezing. If they are still too thick, tweeze a few hairs, one at a time, to thin out.

Thin brows need to be filled in. Use a pencil and a cake brow color, brushed into hairs, to thicken. If you are using a pencil only, fill in and brush pencil lightly into brows. This keeps the penciled brow looking natural.

The shape of your eyes and face dictates the shape of your brows

Here are a few eye and facial shapes that can be corrected with a simple brow shaping:

Close set eyes need to have brows set further apart to make eyes look wider. Start brows about one eighth of an inch beyond inner corner of eye.

Small eyes need a more delicate brow shape. Make brows a bit thinner (but still natural). Make sure to have a good arch, as described above, to help lift and open eyes.

A high forehead requires raised brows. Lift the arch and extend the brow at the ends in a line more straight than curved.

A square face needs curved brows. Focus on the arch and a curved end.

A round face needs brows in a triangular curve, straight at the ends with a high arch in the center.

A narrow forehead can gain width by placing the highest point of the arch further out toward the outer end of the eye.

A very broad forehead should have shortened brows just a quarter of an inch beyond outer corner of the eye. Be careful not to make brows too short for the face.

TIP

A little Coke or Pepsi put in a small bottle and applied with a brush will hold brows in place and won't turn white as hair gel does at times.

All About Brushes

To sculpt and shape features brushes are the must-have tools for the professional artist. That means you!

Brushes are essential for a polished makeup look and the key to correcting and sculpting features. They will make painting your face easier and more fun. Feel brushes for softness—they should be very soft. The best hair types are a natural hair like sable, pony or squirrel, although you should also have a small synthetic brush for applying concealer and eye liner. Some makeup artists are now using large, wide, flat synthetic brushes to apply foundation. It's possible to get a good smooth finish and terrific foundation coverage using this brush.

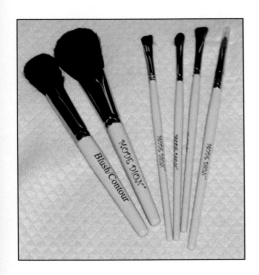

There are a few basic brushes that are essential to every makeup collection:

1. **Large powder brush**—used to set the foundation with loose powder. Be sure hairs are tight together so you have more control. To super-set the foundation, use a puff or sponge and press powder into foundation. Buff excess powder off with the large powder brush for a beautiful, smooth finish.

2. **Cheek contour brush**—used to shape features by following their contours. Smaller than a cheek color brush, some are angled for easier face contouring.

3. **Cheek color brush**—smaller than a powder brush, it is used to add color to the apples of your cheeks. This brush should have rounded plush hairs.

4. **Eye shadow highlighter brush**—this brush is flat and wide. Use it for setting the lids with face powder or for highlighting eyelids and under brows to lift with lightest shadow shade.

5. **Eye shadow defining/contouring brush**—an angled small brush. It is designed for contouring and defining the eye with the darkest shadow color.

6. **Eye shadow balance brush**—the same size as the defining brush but the end is rounded for blending in the edges of the darker shadow color with the medium shadow. This shadow balances eyes to cheeks to lips.

7. **Eye liner brush**—perfect for applying wet/dry liner or liquid liner. They come in sizes from a very skinny, pointy-tipped brush to a thicker pointy tip. The hairs are a bit stiff and firm.

TIP

Long, skinny liner brushes are more difficult to work with. For easier application choose a firmer pointed-tip liner brush.

8. **Brow brush**—a small brush with a firm, slanted or flat top. It is used to apply powder cake brow color or to blend in brow pencil.

9. **Lip brush**—a very important brush used to blend lipstick into lip liner and to create defined edges. Lipstick stays on much better when applying it with this brush. Choose a stiff-tipped brush with shorter hairs for more control. It is a wonderful tool for applying glossy highlighter lipstick. Lip brushes that slide up and down like a periscope last the longest and keep their shape best.

10. **Toothbrush**—keep lips smooth and in top condition by brushing your lips a few times a week. Put a little face wash or lip balm on your lips and brush off all the dead skin that builds up on your lips. Follow with a good lip treatment balm to hydrate the new fresh skin. The benefit? Lipstick goes on easier and lasts longer.

How to wash your makeup brushes

Remember to keep makeup brushes clean. With daily use, wash brushes a few times a month or weekly if you are prone to breakouts.

1) Fill bowl with warm water.
2) Add one squirt of dishwashing liquid or baby shampoo.
3) Swish brushes with water and gently work soap through hairs.
4) Empty water and fill bowl again with fresh warm water.
5) Repeat until water is clear and brushes have no trace of soap.
6) Pat brushes on a dry towel and lay flat on a towel until dry.

When to Say Goodbye

Cosmetics are great tools, but eventually these products, like everything else, get old and should be thrown away. It is not always easy to know when the time has come, so here is a timeline of expiration dates on your favorite basic cosmetic must-haves.

Foundations and moisturizers—can last up to two years, but most last only about a year. When product starts to separate, change consistency or smell funny, it's time to toss it out.

Concealers/coverups—will keep from two to five years until product smells or separates.

Face powder—Loose powder can last three years or more if it doesn't begin to smell funny. Compact powder can harden and turn color as the oil from your skin gets into its surface. Bacteria can build up easily as well. Refresh compact powder and increase its life by scratching off surface layer with a clean toothbrush.

TIPS

Never soak your brushes—the wood will expand and the hairs will fall out.

Never dry brushes standing up because moisture can drip into the base causing it to rot and the hairs will fall out. Never pull on brush hairs, always pat them dry.

Good brushes are an investment that will bring you many years of wonderful use with proper care.

Cheek color—Like a compact powder, bacteria can build up and powder can harden. Treat with the toothbrush technique and keep for two to three years.

Eye shadows—If you keep the top layer clean, these should last up to three years. Look for color changes, bad smells and itchy eyes to point the way to the trash.

Eye liners and lip liners—These can last a long time if you keep them well sharpened. For lip and eye pencils, look for moldy build-up and a change of texture as a throw away signal. Liquid liners last about a year because of a higher risk of bacteria build-up. To keep fresh longer, use a separate clean brush for application instead of the one that goes back into the container.

Mascara—Four months after it has been opened, mascara begins to harbor built-up bacteria that can cause infection and eye irritation. Pumping mascara will push air into the chamber causing it to dry out faster. Stir the wand in the chamber before applying.

Lipstick—After two to three years, color and texture change and bacteria starts to build up.

Face masks (creamy)—will last six months to a year.

Nail polish—two years, give or take.

Fragrance—Not really a beauty tool but an important part of beauty. So the scoop is: keep your fragrance out of sunlight in a dry and cool place. Most people keep their fragrance in the bathroom, which is the worst place of all! Fragrance should last from three to six years if cared for correctly.

How to care for your products and keep them fresh

Store products in a cool, dark place like the refrigerator (cold is a bacteria inhibitor) or a box. Keep out of sunlight and warm, humid places like the bathroom.

- Shake liquids every once in a while. If pigments separate and don't shake back together, toss out the product.

- Avoid touching products with your fingers (because of bacteria). Use sponges, brushes and Q-tips® whenever you can.

- Keep lids closed tightly.

- Never share your products or use those of others.

5
The High Performance Face

Makeup for Stage Lights and Action

From washing out to melting down, stage lights can do a number on your makeup. When creating a makeup look for stage, many performers overcompensate and end up applying too much. Features can become distorted and the look unflattering. Heavy black eye liner drawn around the eyes creates the look of two little black holes. Cheek color overapplied on the apples of the cheeks can look like bright red balls or can turn cheekbones into two red stripes. Lip liner pencil can often be forgotten, creating lipstick so bright you're *all* lips. The makeup color combinations advised in this chapter come from interviews with professional performers from New York to Las Vegas, competition judges, choreographers and convention owners. I asked industry pros their views on the most current and professional combination of shades. The following pages will reveal the perfect performance face, built with neutral colors, to go with every costume and style of performance. The look works as well for smaller stages, competitions or when judges are close to the stage.

To begin your makeup masterpiece, pull your hair back away from your face so your bone structure and features can be easily seen. Make sure you have a good mirror (a magnifying mirror can really help), excellent light, a chair (so you can relax), your makeup at hand and all the tools you will need for a flawless application. You are ready to create your work of art!

The Eyes

When applying performance makeup, remember the importance of balance. The eyes and lips should be balanced—they are the most important on stage since the rest of the face tends to disappear under the lights. Eyes are exaggerated with dark eye shadow, so be careful of under-eye mess from eye shadow fallout. Don't forget the rules: matte or dark shadows pull focus *in* and shimmery or light shadows focus *out*. Matte shadows are best for defining and balancing the eyes under stage lights. For lifting the eyes, light or shimmery shadows are best for the lids and beneath the eyebrows, but do not apply a shimmer shadow over the entire eye area as a base, before adding the matte colors. This will ruin the matte effect and create puffy eyes.

To frame the eyes, some makeup artists like to **define the brows first** before applying eye shadow. This really guides the placement of eye shadow and eye liner. If you need help with brow shaping and placement, check back to page 60 in chapter four. If you already have your brows in check, let's begin!

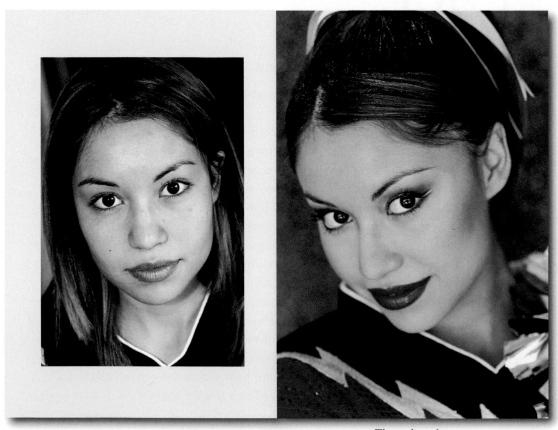

The stadium face

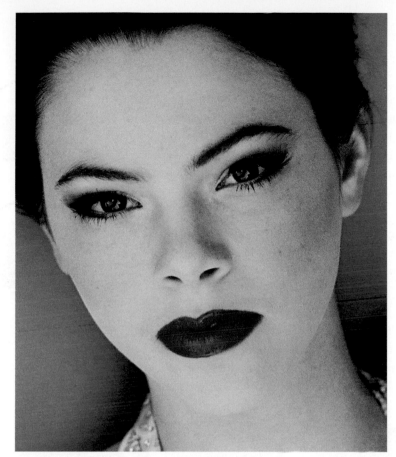

The stage face

Concealer can be oily and cause eye shadow to crease. Use this only if the foundation or shadow base is unable to cover imperfections effectively.

When applying anything to eyelids, lift your chin and lean in close to the mirror. This way, you have a full lid to work on and can see what you are doing clearly.

To find where your dark shadow should end at the outer edge of your eye, use the eyebrow technique. Hold a pencil at the base of the nose pointing to the end of the eyebrow. The pencil's edge along the eye to the end of the brow gives you the outer edge for your shadow. After each application, look straight into the mirror to see if colors are equal on both sides and applied correctly. For more drama and lift, apply matte black shadow from outer corner up to crease and along the crease about a quarter of the way in. Blend into the dark brown shadow shade.

1

After properly using oil-free moisturizer to prevent shine from perspiration, prepare eyelids with a shadow base, foundation or concealer. Make sure to apply across the entire lid from next to the bridge of the nose to the end of eyebrows.

2

Powder eyelid with oil-free loose face powder to create a dry canvas for shadow to go on smoothly. Apply all eye makeup with your eyes open. This will help you easily see the eye crease, so application of the eye shadow and liner will be correct.

3

Define eyes with a dark brown matte shadow. Contour the outer half of the eyelid, blending up just above the eyelid crease. Be sure the shadow lift at the outer eye corner is pointing toward the end of the eyebrow.

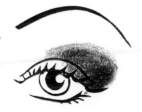

4

Balance eyes with a peachy or red/brown matte shadow to compliment the red tone lip color (an industry standard). Apply it above the crease and across the brow bone, stopping just before the side of the nose. Use this color to blend in edges of the darker shadow for a more polished look.

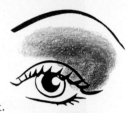

5

Highlight eyes with a cream-color shimmer shadow. Apply onto key points—the inner half of the lid, up under eyebrow and out to the temples.

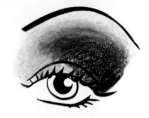

6

Add pop down the center of eye lid, the inner eye corner and brow arch by adding a little sparkling powder. Try gold/white with brown or green eyes or silver/white with blue eyes. This a favorite among pop stars to open and draw attention to eyes.

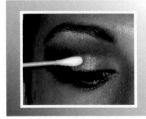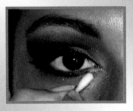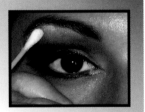

TIP

For beginners using a liquid or wet liner, it can help to first draw a guideline with a pencil or shadow color. Sweep a dry liner brush across shadow color. Brace your right elbow with your left hand for support. Stroke the brush from the outer corner inward. It helps, when first applying any liner, to look straight into the mirror with your eyes wide open to see what the finished effect will be. People see you with your eyes open, not half closed! Always have a supply of Q-tips handy for quick cleanups while liner is still wet. I also like the non-oily eye makeup remover pads. Just be sure the area under eyes is clean before the next step.

7

Line eyes with black cake (wet/dry) or liquid liner. Avoid eye liner pencils because they melt easily under hot conditions. Apply the liner halfway across lid, starting at the outer edge of eye, sweeping up to the crease toward the end of the eyebrow. Then move across the lid, thinning as you go, toward the inner eye corner. Most eyes look best with liner halfway across the upper lid. (For exceptions see chapter four, *Eye Corrections*.) Line lower lashes with brown cake (wet/dry) liner beneath the lashes, sweeping out parallel to above-the-eye crease and end of brow. Do not let the two lines meet. To keep cake liners in place, use eye liner sealer instead of water on the tip of liner brush.

8

Apply white pencil between the upper and lower lines at the outer corner and on the ridge above the lower lash line to create the ultimate *opened* eyes.

The Canvas: Foundation, Concealer & Powder

Whisk away any eye shadow debris. If skin under the eyes is dry, use an eye cream so that concealer will go on smoothly.

Before applying foundation, be sure skin is hydrated with an oil-free moisturizer. (If skin is very dry, use a moisturizer designed for your skin type.) Moisturizer creates a barrier between the foundation and skin; foundation application will be smoother and it will keep your makeup fresh longer.

Blend foundation on forehead, down sides of the nose, sides of face, around the mouth and on lips, chin and jawbone. Finally, blend into the throat. Start with a small amount, gently blending in with clean fingers in downward strokes. The hair on your face grows down, so this will give you the smoothest, most even coverage.

Be sure to blend foundation into the light area under the chin, an area not often tanned by the sun. On stage, when your head is raised, this area can be seen by the audience and looks lighter than the face.

Apply concealer after foundation, otherwise it melts the concealer, taking away some coverage. Use a small synthetic flat brush, a clean lip brush, or your finger to apply. Pat and blend over dark areas at the inner eye corners next to the nose and under the eyes. Apply concealer over areas that foundation cannot cover. Blend edges into foundation for a seamless look.

Set foundation using a large powder brush with loose face powder. If prone to oiliness, choose oil-free loose powder. Blend powder across foundation in downward strokes. (Don't apply much powder under the eye area to avoid dryness and creasing.)

Lips

The eyes are painted, the frame is in place and the canvas set: it is time to balance the face. Lips are the key to balancing your features.

Begin with a freshly sharpened lip pencil. Line lips in red/brown. This pulls lips in at the sides and tones down the red lipstick shade. Line along the outer edge, filling in the lip about halfway in. Turn your head to the side to make sure lips appear full and can be easily seen from that angle.

Apply red lipstick with a lip brush (for longer-lasting coverage) to evenly pull the lips forward with color. I find a creamy opaque color holds up best and is less drying than a matte finish.

Create *showstopper* lips with a shimmer lip highlighter, either lip gloss or lipstick. Apply at the centers of upper and lower lips to add light-catching pop.

TIPS

Choose a concealer color that's about half a shade lighter than your foundation, with a little yellow in it. For facial imperfections, try a blemish treatment concealer that covers and heals.

For a *super set*, apply powder to a puff or cotton square and gently press powder all over into foundation. With a large powder brush, buff off excess powder and smooth out the finish.

Fill in lips with a lip pencil to make lipstick last longer. Pencils increase staying power —when lipstick starts to fade, the pencil remains, providing color. Look one step ahead as you draw, a little like riding a bike or driving a car.

For super staying power, apply pencil and lipstick. Place tissue over lips and using a large brush, dust powder over tissue. The powder helps the tissue pull out excess oil and seals color. You can also use a lipstick sealer. Often used for kissing scenes in movies, this clear liquid seals on the lip color without drying out lips.

Brows Frame the Masterpiece

Some makeup artists like to apply brows after the canvas has been prepped—after foundation, concealer and powder to give your brows maximum definition and shape. Foundation and powder can get into the brow hairs and need to be brushed out. There are two choices of brow defining tools: the dry cake color and the pencil liner color.

Dry cake color requires a small angled brush or a pointy brush to apply color. These are good for making brows look thicker and filling in bare areas.

The pencil liner can shape and define, but should be brushed out a bit to look more natural. Brow brushes blend color into the brow hair and kind of shred the pencil color, making it look like hairs. To create a thin brow, draw a line one shade darker through the center of the brow. Blend foundation and face powder over brow hairs to cover around the line. On stage this creates the illusion that brows are thinner than they really are.

Create Bone Structure & Add Liveliness to the Face with Cheek Color

To contour your cheeks, choose a pinkish brown color. Look for a neutral color about three shades darker than your own skin. Use this shade to define your bone structure (see *Face Physics, Correcting and Shaping Features*, page 53) and to shade your cheekbones. With your finger, feel along the underside of your cheekbone. Apply color from the center of your ear, blend along the bone toward the base of your nostrils. Stop two fingers out from your nose and sweep color up like a hook around cheek apples.

To flush cheeks, choose a soft red or rose color. This will compliment the red lip shade used for the stage. Apply blush sparingly with a cheek brush to the apples of the cheeks up to the cheekbones in a teardrop shape and a little on the sides of the forehead.

For high cheekbones, use a sparkling shimmer powder with a brush. Tap off excess so it is applied lightly, then dust high on cheekbones to the temples.

Lashes Go Last

Most performers wear false lashes. If you choose to wear them, apply mascara after they have been secured. For a high-energy performance, when perspiration and athletic movements are involved, the best choice is to use mascara only. Perspiration loosens false lashes, and vigorous athletic movements can knock them off. Instead of having to worry about your lashes, not to mention your eyesight, use three coats of mascara to open eyes. Apply black mascara—no matter what your hair color is.

The truth about false lashes

Size

False lashes vary in size from short (just enough to bring out your eyes) to long for deluxe drama. Human hair lashes are the most comfortable, hold up well and can be used several times. Individual lashes are little clusters glued on just where you feel a bit more lash is needed, but these can be harder to use than an entire strip of lashes. For the stage, try thicker strips. Consider the best size for your performance style. Try natural lashes for ballet or for a slight enhancement and super length for cabaret and funk.

The cut

Most lashes need trimming. To make sure you have the right fit, place the false lash along your lash line. It should stop about one-eighth of an inch away from the inner eye corner. Cut them down to size by snipping off the longer outer end. Be sure to save that piece for natural outer eyelash extensions later.

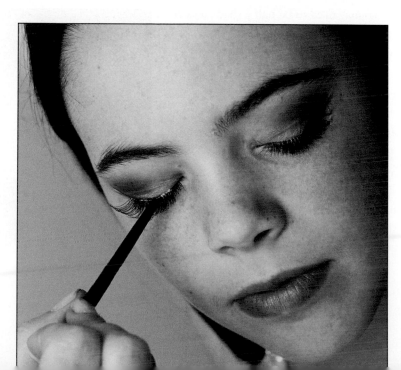

TIP

For more open eyes always curl lashes first. Curl once near the roots, at the center, and then again near the end of the lashes. Before applying mascara, wipe the wand with a tissue to clean off the excess that could cause clumping. Do the bottom lashes first, keeping the brush on its side and rubbing back and forth. Go to the top lashes and do the same, starting at the roots of the lashes and rubbing side to side as you work out to the end of the lashes. The side-to-side rub separates lashes and helps to distribute mascara evenly. Focus on the outer corner of the lashes. A lash comb is helpful to have just in case of clumps and is very useful when using false lashes, too. Never pump wand in and out of mascara tube. This draws air into the chamber and causes the mascara to dry out.

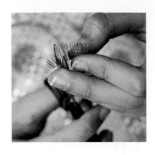

TIP

Apply false lashes after eye shadow and liner. The false lashes can block your view, making it harder to see close up, and makeup can collect in them. False lashes that have lost their curl can be brought back to life by gently curling them with an eyelash curler.

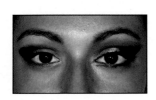

The stick

Use clear lash glue (it comes in black or clear). The clear is white coming out of the tube but dries clear so that even if you make a mistake it won't ruin your makeup. Squeeze a small amount of glue across the base of lash or onto a tissue for dipping. Now count to ten so the glue can dry a bit and become tacky. Apply lash at the roots of your own lashes. Start at outer corner. Glue on lash just at the outer edge of eye corner. Look in the mirror and check lash position. If it looks right (not too far in or out), you are ready to secure across the root line. Hold tips of the false lash and press in as you go across. Glue will stick to your fingertips, so use the end of a makeup brush or tweezers to push lashes into place. For individual lashes, place one cluster at a time, starting at the outer corner. Use tweezers to hold onto the lashes and help with placement.

Apply one light coat of mascara. Create a seamless look by starting at the roots of your real lashes at the inner most eye corner, blending mascara into lashes across to outer eye corner.

Makeup for Large Theaters, Recitals & Large Productions

There are times a stronger look is needed. When there is a lot of distance between the performer and the audience these areas of the face need more enhancing:

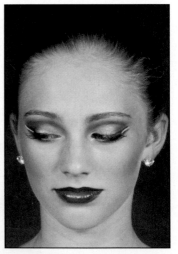

- Brows may need to be half a shade darker than hair color for brunettes, and all brows will need extra focus by lengthening the outer end.

- For more definition apply the dark brown defining shadow three-quarters of the way across the eye bone just above the crease.

- To intensify eyes, black shadow can be applied at the outer corner of the eyes stopping just above the crease extending toward the end of the brows. Blend into the edges of the brown shade halfway across into the crease.

Makeup Application for the Junior Performer

A junior performer usually is a preteen, and can be as young as four years old. They have smaller, more delicate features than their teen/adult counterparts. A lighter application is necessary to keep them looking their age and not overpower their features. In most cases, juniors do not apply their own makeup. A mother or an assigned makeup artist will undertake this task, which can sometimes prove quite challenging. Juniors are not accustomed to having someone poke around their eyes, and hate sitting still for any length of time! Mascara, liner and lipstick can prove particularly difficult. Here are a few easy techniques that have worked well for me to keep your junior looking great and feeling more comfortable.

Just as for any makeup application, it is important to *prepare the skin*. Clean with a face wash (soap is drying and can sting eyes) and follow with an oil-free moisturizer. Teaching good skin care is important even at the youngest of ages especially for those who perspire more heavily.

Shape and define brows to frame the eyes. The look of the brows is extremely important for the young performer. Most juniors have messy brows because they are not yet old enough to tweeze. Complete brow color before eye color. Fill in along the center of brow with brow cake on a pointed brush or use a brow pencil.

When you begin color application on the junior face *do the eyes first*. Any debris or smudging that occurs can be easily cleaned up after application. Powder eyelids

TIP

Before approaching the young performer with shadow on a brush, use your finger and stroke the eyelid where shadow will be applied, explaining " I will be applying a little color here just like the big girls do, ok?" This prepares her for the feeling, and she will not be startled or afraid.

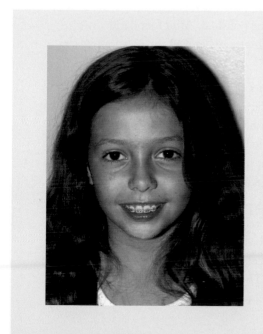
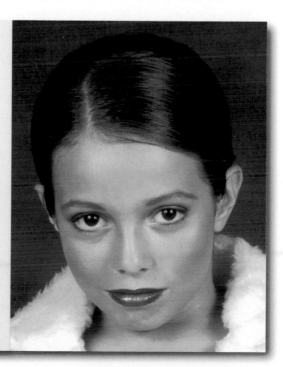

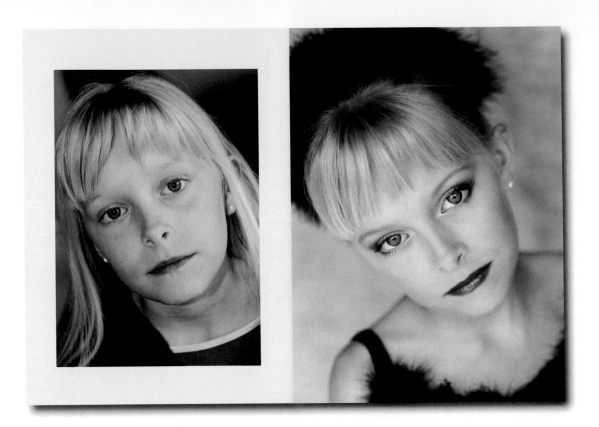

with loose face powder so shadow goes on smoothly. If lids show veins or freckles, cover first with foundation and set with powder.

Creating the canvas: even a young dancer with perfect skin needs to apply a light foundation. Facial skin flushes while performing, especially down the front of the face which effects the cheek color. A thin cover of oil-free foundation (over moisturizer) keeps the red in check and the face looking polished. After foundation, use concealer in a golden tone to cover dark circles under eyes if needed, then set makeup with translucent face powder.

Lips: To keep lips still, have junior close her lips. Line lips with a red/brown lip liner. Keep lips rounded at the top and wide at the sides. Be sure lips can be seen in profile. Fill in with lip liner. Juniors have small lips—and lipsticks are too large to apply directly. Using a sheer red tone, apply lipstick with a lip brush, shaping lips and blending into the lip pencil. Highlight lips at center of lower and upper lip with a little glossy or shimmery lipstick to soften the red tone and create fullness.

A flush on the apples of the cheeks with a sheer red cheek tone is just enough to warm the face. Have junior smile wide to find the rounds of the cheeks. Before applying, tap off excess cheek color from brush on a tissue so the application is softer. Using a contour color to define cheekbones, nose line and chin on a junior is optional and should be done sparingly. This is best used for a large theater production, where features can become washed out.

With the junior's eyes open:

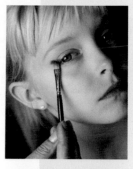

1 **Define outer corner** of eye with matte brown shadow, blending just above eye crease, up and halfway into the eye bone. Applying with eyes open helps you see the stopping point, slightly above the crease, at the end of the eye, toward the end of the eyebrow. Next, fill in at outer corner lash line and then up across the outer half of eye bone, just above crease with eyes closed. Make sure to keep three-quarters of the inner lid free from the brown shadow.

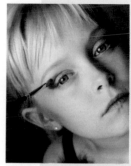

2 **Balance eyes** with a peach or red/brown color eye shadow. Blend across eye bone just above crease, stopping just before the brow begins. Blend in edges to soften the color.

3 **Highlight eyelid** and under brow with cream shimmer shadow.

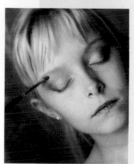

4 **Open eyes** with a sparkling shimmer powder just at the center of eyelid, at inner eye corners and at arch of brow. If arch is not apparent, this will create one. This can really make a difference when seen from a distance.

5 **Line eyes** using a firm pointy liner brush with brown wet/dry cake eyeliner. (Liquid liner takes too long to dry, so younger performers can easily smudge it, and pencil liners don't last through long performances and can be rubbed off easily.) Begin under lower lashes. Wet brush with water or eye liner sealer liquid (good for teary eyes). Stir into the brown shadow cake liner until creamy, tap off excess and begin at the outer corner of the lower lash line, blending out just beyond the eye crease at the end of the eye. Instruct junior to look up towards the ceiling and focus on something.

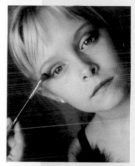

While lining her eyes tell junior "Almost done! See how easy?" Juniors like to know the end of the ordeal is near (even if it's not). Avoid saying things like "Don't move! Hold still, wait a minute!" With her eyes wide open, use black shadow cake liner, starting at outer corner of upper lid, sweeping liner up towards end of brow, stopping just beyond eye crease. Do not let the brown and black lines meet. Do not line upper lid. To make it easier, try a dry run this way: before wetting brush, swipe dry liner brush across cake liner and try to get perfect lines. If it looks good, wet brush and follow your dry lines. Be sure junior sits up straight, lifts her chin slightly and looks away from the direction you're working. Apply a soft white pencil between the brown and black lines at the outer eye corner to open the eyes—making sure pencil is freshly sharpened. If white pencil is too hard, run tip under warm water to soften, then dry and apply to eyes.

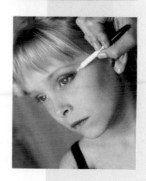

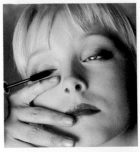

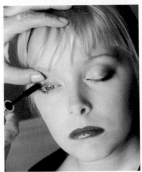

Use black mascara on lashes even for those with blonde hair—it really opens the eyes. Mascara can be very difficult to apply on a junior. First, clean off excess mascara from the wand with tissue. Ask the junior to look up to the ceiling, place your little finger under lower lashes then wiggle the mascara on lower lashes and your finger. Quickly say "Done!" (That way, mascara gets on your finger, not her face.) Next, have her look straight ahead and slightly down. Suggest something for her to focus on. Tilt her chin slightly and place your thumb gently on eyelid, slightly lifting lid to clear the lash line. Apply mascara at inner corner then outer corner, from roots out, wiggling from side to side as you go. Make sure junior keeps her chin up and focus down, away from application area. False lashes can be applied to juniors, but it is best to cut them in half, applying the small side to the outer half of the lash line.

When performing in a large theater, eye liner can be applied across half of the upper lid and below lower lashes. Lipstick can be darkened to opaque red. Facial contouring and slightly stronger cheek color can also help enhance facial features.

Makeup for Deep Skin Tones

Makeup shades, when used on a deeper skin tones, require stronger pigment colors. Application instructions are described above, but colors are stronger on eyes, cheeks and lips.

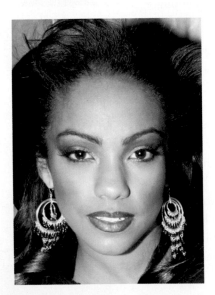

To enhance and add drama to the eyes:

- Define at outer corner with black eye shadow, blending up to eye crease and across eye bone half way in. Create more definition with a deep brown shadow, blending into the edges of the black shadow across eye bone.

- Add red/brown or burgundy eye shadow across eye bone out to the end of brows.

- Highlight lid and under brow with beige/gold shimmer shadow.

- Line eyes with the application described previously, but use black liquid liner for more intensity across upper and lower lash line. Remember to keep liner apart at outer eye corner and apply white pencil between the lines and onto lower lid ridge.

- Use thick black false lashes to bring out and open eyes.

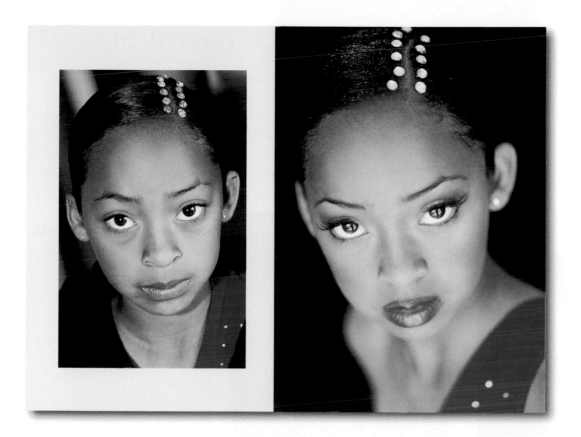

It is important for brows to stand out against deeper skin tones.

Lips and cheeks need a richer tone.

- Line lips using a deep brown (natural) or burgundy/red (stage) and blend. Lip shade should be a strong red or burgundy. Pop color at the center of the upper and lower lip with a highlighter.
- Use a blush in a deep burgundy red and contour with a deep brown/red to enhance features. Ebony skin should use a dark brown contour color.

TIP

Strong pigments require you to focus even more on blending. Make sure to tap off excess color from makeup brushes before applying and blend well the edges of one color into the next.

Beauty on the Pageant Stage

Many performers enjoy competing in beauty pageants. From Miss USA to local pageants, the best way to know what makeup look is expected is to follow the guidelines provided by credible organizations. How much and what style of makeup to apply varies greatly, from polished, soft looks to full stage makeup. Usually the director of the pageant will tell the judges what makeup style to look for. Most prefer a look that shows up well on stage, is age appropriate and compliments the beauty of the contestant. When in doubt, research past contest winners and check out their style.

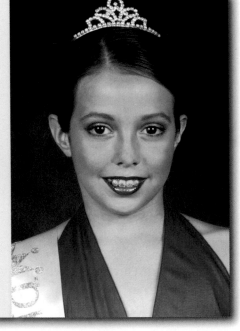

After many interviews with pageant professionals including Carl Dunn, CEO of *Pageantry* magazine (the oldest in the business) and Blair Griffith, winner of Miss Congeniality at the Miss Teen USA pageant, I got the scoop on the polished pageantry face.

All ages on stage

All pageant contestants need to enhance brows, eyes, facial features, lashes (false lashes in *natural* for the teen or adult), cheek color and lipstick. Shimmer is popular on cheekbones, key light-catching areas of the eyes and on exposed areas of the body. *But glitter is to be avoided!* Makeup should not be a distraction. Makeup and hair changes are encouraged for each look (if there is time) and should compliment your features as well as your dress or costume style. If there is time for a makeup change, sporty or swimsuit looks should be more natural and evening/gown makeup should be more glamorous. Use hairpieces for quick-change looks. Make sure your nails are properly groomed and in a soft neutral color.

Youth

Ages six to nine should have soft makeup. For an interview, a no-makeup look is the norm. This means clear lip gloss, brows shaped, and blemishes covered (see *No Makeup Rule*, page 84 in this chapter). In the talent and formal category, more makeup can be applied, as in *Makeup Application for the Junior Performer*, page 73. Some pageants prefer a slightly lighter eye liner, cheek color, and lipstick application but remember to be careful your makeup look doesn't fade under stage lights. For a soft look that will show from the stage, try a soft peach or pink lip color with a complimentary cheek shade, or try the peach or pink over a sheer red. A natural color lip liner paired with red lipstick can soften the look too. Use a lip liner to insure softer lip colors won't fade.

Casual looks should have soft, sheer glossy lips, a soft flush to the cheeks and light eye shadow without noticeable eyeliner.

Teen to adult

For the interview, follow the steps covered in *Daylight Pageant Makeup* in chapter three. For stage/formal, follow the steps covered in this chapter *Makeup for Large Theaters, Recitals & Large Productions*. For pageants like Miss Teen USA, which prefer a softer stage face, change the colors a bit.

Instead of using red/brown or peachy eye shadow color to balance eyes to lips, try a beige/brown so the eyes are more neutral. Instead of red lipstick try a sheer lipstick in rose, pink, or red/burgundy. (Adult contestants can always get away with more dramatic makeup and often need a stronger lipstick shade to add life to the face.) Make sure your eye liner does not meet at the corners and avoid long eye liner extensions, used in the performance face look. A white pencil on

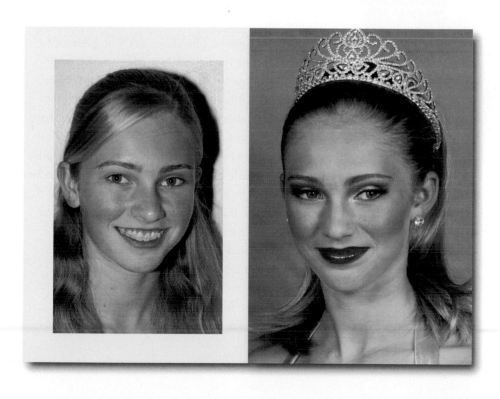

TIP

Don't be afraid to layer colors. Try a peach lipstick with a pink gloss, or a red lipstick with a gold gloss. Even nail polish can look beautiful layered. It's fun to create your own colors and play with what looks good against your skin, eyes and hair color.

the ridge above the lower lashes, will open eyes. Remember the rule: the darker the eyes, the lighter the lips. *Radiance* is important in pageantry so be sure to add a gloss for shine. Shimmer is beautiful on the cheekbones and eyes as well as exposed skin for a more glamorous look. Blending is vital! The judges sit close to the stage.

For a casual/swimsuit presentation (if you have time to adjust your makeup) go soft on the lips opting for glossy beige/pinks or peach with a pink/brown lip liner. Eyeliner should be natural looking in brown or plum, not black.

Backstage with Blair

Blair Griffith, winner of "Miss Congeniality" in Miss Teen USA 2006 and a former Miss Teen Colorado, suggests keeping makeup soft (the *Teen to adult* interview look, page 79). Since many of the Miss USA contestants are interviewed in everything from professional suits and dresses to casual trendy clothing, makeup should complement the style.

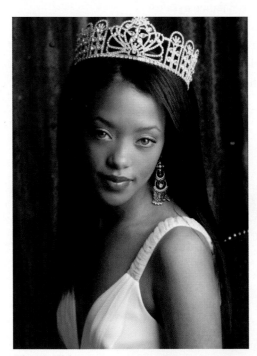

Blair Griffith

Contestants are expected to do their own hair and makeup—a professional makeup artist does a quick touch-up before going on stage. An appropriate teen look is to have glossy lips in soft pink or beige with a natural lip liner. The lighter lip look is paired with stronger eyes as shown in our stage look. Many pop stars like this combination as well. Remember the rule: stronger eyes, lighter lips, except for the *theme* performance looks, shown in chapter seven. This does vary from pageant to pageant. A red tone lipstick with a red/brown lip liner shows up better under stage lights and is still a standard in many pageants. Blair's makeup artist touched up her look with navy eyeliner. She loved the way her eyes stood out with a little more color but still looked natural. This is an easy way to add color to eyes without using a bright eye shadow. She only lined the top lid and kept the under eyeliner a natural brown. Of course, the most versatile eye liner colors are the neutrals shown on page 79. Blair learned two beauty secrets: drink lots of water to stay hydrated and it should a pimple pop up, put a little mouthwash on it. Clean breath and a clear face—what more could a pageant beauty ask for!

When wearing a banner, remember to keep your hair off your shoulders, even when worn down. Many contestants like to wear their hair up or in a side ponytail for this reason.

Extreme Condition Beauty

For performers who are exposed to very hot, cold or wet environments, makeup has to be set to last. Whether ice skating, marching in a parade or cheering to the crowds, looking your best means using products that are oil-free, moisture resistant and designed with stronger pigments. These tips will help:

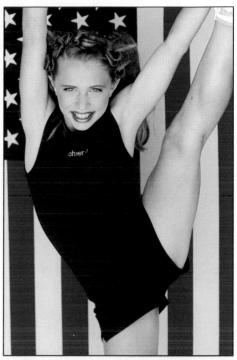

Extreme heat

Avoid highly fragranced formulations and perfumes. Heat can increase potential for irritation. The sun, combined with fragrance, can cause skin discoloration. Use products that contain mint, which has a long-lasting cooling effect on the skin. When performing out in the sun always use an oil-free sunscreen, at least SPF 25, under makeup for protection. If you become red or inflamed, either from heat rash or sun exposure, use products that contain aloe vera to soothe. Be sure to use a lip balm with SPF protection under lipstick, as lips are first to burn.

Use oil-free products. Anything that goes on your face, including cleanser, moisturizer (a must to hold makeup), foundations and powders, should be oil-free even if your skin is a bit dry. Excess oils will only break down your makeup and take away staying power. If skin is on the oily side, look for products labeled "oil-control."

Use products with rich pigments. Skip any product that says sheer or light. Stay way from shadows and cheek colors with shimmer, as they will only make you look oily. Use products that can be used wet or dry, a sure sign of rich pigments.

Set makeup. Use a lipstick sealer to hold lip color and eye liner sealer to make eyeliner waterproof. Set lids before eye color with an eye shadow base or powder. Avoid oily concealers.

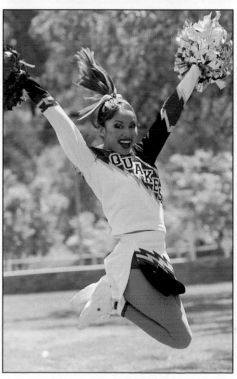

Waterproof your lashes. Use waterproof mascara on lashes and skip fake lashes when you're exposed to extreme heat and moisture.

Makeup on ice

Ice skating has specific makeup challenges. Hot spotlights can wash out your makeup look, and reflection off the ice onto your face can create shadows. Because of the lighting in ice rinks, *cool undertone* lips, cheeks and eyes can make you look tired. It's best to follow the basic stage rules we've covered using neutrals with slightly warmer tones. If you want brighter *cool* color tones on the eyes, choose gray instead of blue or plum instead of purple. If you love pink on cheeks and lips, be careful to choose warmer pinks over cool, more violet pinks. The basic stage face we have described in this chapter works well for ice skating, but the glamorous costumes and sparkling ice will require a few little touches:

Shimmer powder is ideal for performances on ice. Opaque shimmer powder in a white gold or white silver tone will bring out your features and provide radiance. Place shimmer powder in the key light-catching points: inner eye corners (to address under eye dark shadows), the brow arch to lift eyes, the center of lid to draw attention to your gaze and a light dusting high on the cheekbones.

Glitter spray applied to the hair, shoulders, chest and back (if exposed) can draw attention to the body as you move.

Loose glitter in soft colors like opal/pastel, a white sparkle, applied lightly to center of lips can be beautiful with glitzy costuming. Apply sparingly, and be sure to seal glitter on the face.

False lashes really help eyes look wide and open. Remember, the look you want is elegant and beautiful, not overdone.

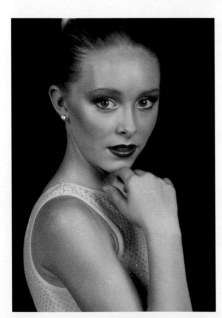

Pull hair back and smooth, avoiding the use of bobby pins and hair rhinestones, as they are a hazard on the ice. French braids are good if hair is layered and look very pretty with a ribbon woven through them.

Show choir

With non-stop performing—up to thirty minutes of singing, dancing and dazzling audiences—they bring new meaning to quick change and high energy. That's why Show Choir falls into the *extreme condition* performing. The performance face covered in this chapter will suit your needs perfectly. Remember, keep your look elegant, sophisticated and polished. Avoid makeup that is too bright or overdone. With so many fast changes, try to vary your look a little with each costume. When using glitter, have a roll of first aid tape for quick glitter removal between changes (see *Glitter, dazzling or dangerous?*, page 86). Hairpieces and wigs will add excitement and help keep you looking fresh for each number.

Cheer, color guard, drill, twirl and band

Uniforms in school colors create team spirit. For multiple costume and uniform changes it is best to stay with the neutral performance face. But for brighter, more lively makeup that complements such school colors as blue and teal or burgundy and purple, try these easy color themes. Follow the performance face application technique making these adjustments:

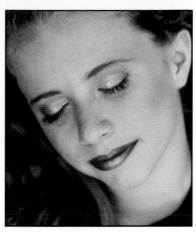

Makeup for blues

To complement blues and other cool colors: define eyes with a deep navy matte shadow. To balance eyes above crease and across eye bone use a matte medium neutral gray. Highlight eyes with a sheer white or silver shimmer shadow. Keep lips in a red tone but highlight at the center with a glossy white shimmer lipstick.

To complement purple and burgundy colors: define eyes with a deep plum/purple matte. Balance eyes with a burgundy/rose matte shadow. Highlight with a pink shimmer or silver shadow. Lips should be a burgundy red with burgundy lip liner. Highlight at the center with a glossy pink shimmer lipstick.

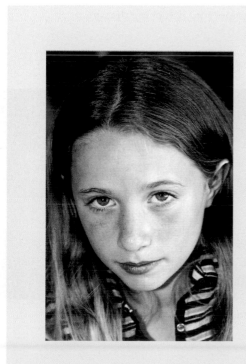

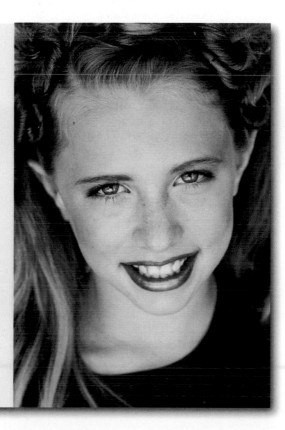

Dealing With the "No Makeup" Rule

Some performers, like gymnasts or cheerleaders, might be asked to have a *no makeup* look. Of course, you still want to look your best and if a few minor imperfections have you worried, remember—just don't let them see your flaws.

That means finding a *perfect* skin tone match in a foundation and powder. Apply foundation to even out skin and cover breakouts, then set it with a little powder to control shine. Cover dark under eye circles so you won't look tired, and blend carefully so it's undetectable. Follow the brow rules by defining, arching and naturally extending to create a natural-looking frame to your eyes. Curl lashes and apply mascara lightly to help open eyes, then use a lash comb to separate clumps. Apply a natural pinky-beige cheek color, if needed, to add just a slight hint of flush to apples of cheeks. Apply the same color on the brow bone to warm the eyes. Highlight eyes on lids and under eyebrows with a light matte eye shadow, to accent lids and lift eyes. If lips are small, line them slightly fuller at the sides with a lip pencil the same shade as your lip color, and apply clear or natural colored lip gloss that's not sticky.

Now you understand all the effort that goes into achieving that *no makeup* look!

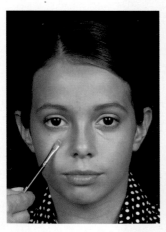
Conceal

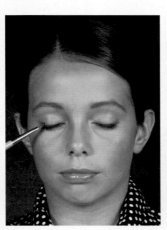
Soft eyes

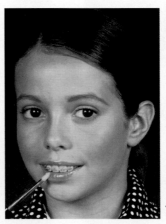
Natural gloss

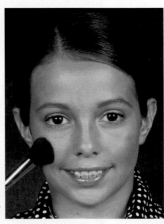
Soft cheeks

Checklist:
the Performer's Makeup Bag

Makeup

- foundation
  concealer
  loose powder
  eye shadow base
  eye shadow*
  white pencil
  mascara
  lipstick
  lip liner
  shimmer powder
  false lashes
  lash glue
  highlighter

* Four eye shadow
  colors: matte black,
  matte brown, matte
  peach or red/brown
  and cream color
  shimmer. Good
  pigments will allow
  the use of shadows
  as a wet or dry eye
  liner too. These
  four colors are
  neutral and go with
  all costumes.

Other necessities

- Band-Aids®
  safety pins
  feminine products
  aspirin
  antacids
  breath mints
  deodorant
  extra tights
  paper and pen
  hair brush
  hair spray
  bobby pins
  Scotch tape
  first aid tape
    (for roaming glitter)
  socks
  foot powder
  body lotion
  nail clipper/file
  nail polish remover

- eye makeup remover pad
  (non-oily is best)

- small scissors
  *Use this handy tool for trimming false
  lashes and cutting hanging threads.*

- tweezers
  *Eye makeup looks its best when the
  brows are well groomed, to remove stray
  hairs. Also use tweezers to perfectly
  place rhinestones.*

- eyelash curler
  *For perfectly curled lashes. Always curl
  lashes before you put on mascara or false
  lashes, never after.*

- cosmetic pencil sharpener
  *Lip and white eye pencils must have a
  perfect point.*

- cotton squares and swabs
  *Wet cotton squares with warm water
  and a little face wash to do a fast clean-up
  without even needing a towel.*

- Q-tips
  *Great to spot-clean quickly, removing
  mascara smudges or eye shadow flecks.*

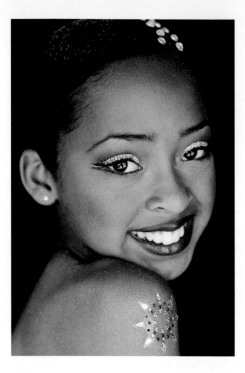

Go For Glitter
& Glitz With Style

Products

Here are a few more quick add-on products to pump up the volume of show appeal:

Glitter tattoos come in all colors and designs. Wear on your face or body to add exotic flair to your look.

Highlighting shimmer powder: a performer's best friend. Shimmering powder sets off your skin, highlights your features and gives a beautiful radiance to your look. Apply *opaque* shimmer to center of lids, under brows and at inner eye corners. Use sheer shimmer on cheekbones, shoulders, chest and any exposed skin you want to show off.

Glitter body gel: Use where you want to draw attention and highlight. It can also be used to seal on glitter—just pat loose glitter on top of wet gel and glitter will stay on.

Glitter spray: For hair, body and costume, it's easy to use and perfect for applying to large areas adding radiance under lights. Be sure to spray at least a foot away from the target area so the glitter can be applied evenly.

Rhinestones can be any size from tiny little accents to large shimmering stones. To apply, make dots with an eye pencil in the spot you want for the rhinestone. Squeeze little drops of eyelash glue onto marks, and wait a minute for glue to get tacky. Using tweezers, grip rhinestone and place flat side down in glue. These provide the ultimate twinkle. (Also see page 117.)

Glitter: *dazzling or dangerous? Use it right!*

When used correctly, glitter can be beautiful, add show appeal and be a wonderful complement to costumes and uniforms. Follow these application rules and *face physics* (page 53) to look your very best. Glitter is for key light-catching points and is powerful, so use it sparingly. Here is everything you need to know:

Loose glitter: Look for flat-cut glitter, not grainy, which is hard to keep on. Avoid glitter mixed with powder because it can look crusty when sealed on. For a beautiful, glitzy smile, pat glitter onto lips in shades like red, pink or burgundy.

To seal glitter on: Lip gloss, Vaseline, cream adhesive (found in glitter crayons or tube products) and hairspray (the worst), will not only cause rashes and irritation, but melt the minute a performer gets hot and begins to perspire. To hold glitter on tight, use water-soluble spirit gum or glitter gel that dries water-resistant. To use correctly, spread a thin application onto any area where glitter is to be applied, using a Q-tip or small brush. Allow adhesive to dry a few seconds, until tacky. Dip the wet end of the Q-tip or brush into the loose glitter so it sticks, then pat it on to adhesive until the desired amount is in place. With a clean face brush, dust off any glitter particles, especially around the eyes, that might not have been sealed. You don't want glitter in your eyes or moving around!

Use glitter only in key light-catching points: Avoid over-doing the glitter look. The key light catching points are: cheekbones, eye temples, high on eye bones, brow arches, inner eye corners and center of eyelids. Glitter can look great on center of the upper and lower lip or lightly pressed into lipstick.

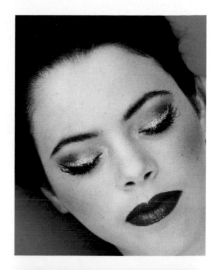

Get rid of roving glitter: Glitter that's fallen onto the face can't be rubbed off. You can easily remove those roving particles with first aid tape. Choose the "gentle paper" first aid tape for facial use. Place tape over glitter, press gently, and slowly peel away. It is also perfect for quick changes, when one number calls for glitter and the next doesn't. Your shadow and lipstick stays perfect, and there is minimal, if any, touch-up needed.

To remove: Remember, when removing eye glitter and makeup, cleanse, swiping eyes in downward strokes, not side-to-side, as this works the glitter and eye makeup into your eyes.

Contact lenses and glitter

Those with contacts have a hard time with products like false lashes and glitter. Putting contacts in before applying makeup can prevent it from getting in under the lens. If you are very sensitive to working around the eye, try putting contacts in last, after all makeup is on, but use eye drops first to be sure eyes are clean.

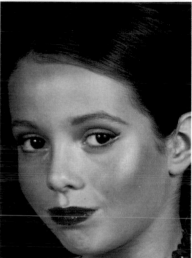

Glitter themes

Red glitter looks great on the lips for glitzy jazz or tap numbers. Silver glitter on the center of eyelids can look like rhinestones and add glamour. White opalescent glitter on the lips or face looks ethereal and elegant. Choose glitter that's appropriate for the theme.

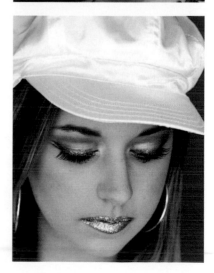

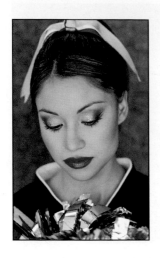

Sport glitter

Over-the-top spirit-themed glitter, layered in a row up the eyelids in the uniform or school colors, is more of a carnival look. If you want to be creative using your spirit colors, be sure you still follow *face physics* (page 53) to enhance your features. Silver or light colored glitter on the eye bone just above the crease makes eyes look puffy. Only use highlighting colors on key light-catching points. Red or pink glitter close to the eyes can make them look bloodshot. Eyes lined with long glitter extensions, out to eye temples, can make eyes look small and overdone. Don't be lazy with your makeup application and use glitter *in place* of eye shadow! Glitter should be used on top of correctly applied eye shadow. Glitter, when used alone, does nothing but make eyes look puffy and small. Many competition judges at dance and cheer events have said how they would love to see spirited, yet flattering, makeup looks.

Getting glitter in your eyes by wearing too much can cause discomfort and the possibility of injury. Many competitions have banned its use because of these concerns. Stunt performers should be especially cautious.

Glitter stenciling

Glitter stencils are a great way to create fun sparkling fantasy designs that are easy to apply. At any craft store you will find a variety of stencils in many different designs and sizes. Choose the design that goes best with your theme. Cut out around your stencil so it is easy to work with. Place stencil on skin and using a Q-tip or small makeup brush, evenly apply water-soluble spirit gum or glitter gel sealer in the stencil. Dip applicator into glitter and pat into stencil. Pull away stencil and there you have it, a perfect design!

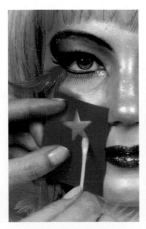
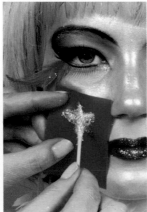
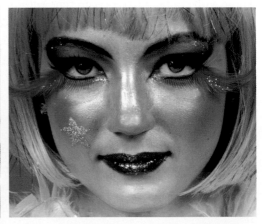

Ten Makeup Mistakes Never to Make on Stage

You might have all the right moves, but your makeup could give you away as still being an amateur. Industry professionals point to these common mistakes:

1 Too washed out ∽
Under the bright lights of stage or video, your coloring and features can fade. Wear a foundation that matches your body, not your face. Blend it down onto your throat so it looks natural. Make sure to sculpt the sides of your nose, cheekbones and even the jaw line if needed.

2 Too shiny ∽
Let your talent shine, not your face. Keep makeup long lasting by powdering after foundation and on eyelids before shadow. Use oil-free moisturizer.

3 Undefined brows ∽
Brows are the frame to your eyes and balance your face. Use a brow pencil or brow cake to shape and define.

4 Black eye liner all around the eye ∽
Black liner applied all around eyes from corner to corner closes the eyes and from a distance makes eyes look like two little black holes. Always keep the corners of the eye open where the top and bottom liner meet.

5 Out of style shadow looks ∽
Blue shadow was a stage standard in the past, but just as fashion changes, so does makeup. Today, professionals look for a more natural look that doesn't overpower the features. Unless your choreographer or director asks for blue shadow, stay with brown and gray tones.

6 Invisible lashes ∽
Learn to use false lashes. The pros know these make your eyes come alive.

7 Messy lips ∽
Learn to use a lip liner and shape your lips. This prevents running and holds lip color too.

8 No lips or all lips ∽
Lips can disappear with only lip gloss or become too big with overly bright lip colors. Red/brown lip liners pull lips in and brighter lipstick on top pulls lips out. Highlighter lipstick pops the center of lips forward. Build your lips to perfection!

9 The wrong makeup theme ∽
Don't come in bold dramatic makeup when you're dancing a classical ballet or performing a street-style piece. Juniors should always wear age-appropriate makeup for performances.

10 Lack of knowledge ∽
Learn the craft of good makeup application. Experiment, practice and ask advice from experts. Everyone loves to share tips! You can learn a lot from the pros—listen to them.

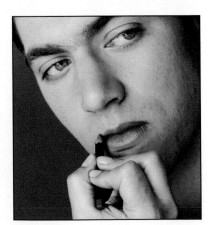

Define brows

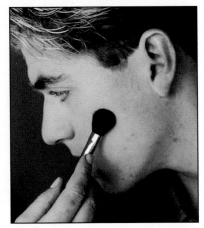

Contour features

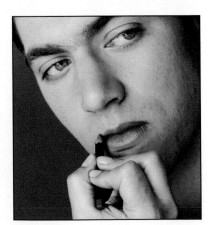

Define lips

Makeup for Men

Stage lights can wash out even the most sculpted faces. For men, makeup can be a great asset to even out skin color and define features. The needs of the man and what he is performing will dictate how much makeup is required. The following guidelines will give you an idea of when and where a little help is needed.

Standard makeup for men

- Cleanse skin before warming up or performing and thoroughly remove makeup and perspiration after every performance to avoid breakouts. Before using foundation to even the skin tone, it's important to apply an oil-free moisturizer to keep skin smooth and help makeup last.

- Apply a thin layer of oil-free foundation to prevent redness from hot lights and exertion to even out skin color and conceal breakouts. Be sure to use a golden/yellow undertone foundation to look more natural.

- Conceal under-eye darkness with yellow tone concealer. Use only where needed. To apply the least amount of concealer with the maximum coverage, use a synthetic concealer brush.

- Set foundation and keep shine in check with a light dusting of translucent face powder.

- Contour and define features such as cheekbones, along the sides of the nose, center of chin or along jawbone using a pinky/brown cheek color.

- Shape brows and fill in where needed with brow pencil or brow cake color to frame eyes.

- Tweeze out or trim unruly brow hairs. Comb brows, sideburns and other facial hair where needed.

- Fill in an uneven lip line with lip pencil in a flesh tone pinky/brown color the same color as lips. Intense workouts cause dehydration, which can chap lips. Use a lip balm to keep lips in top condition.

- Mascara in brown can help bring out blonde or fair eye lashes.

In a large theater

- Define eyes along lash line at outer half of eye with brown cake liner. Use eyeliner sealer to prevent running. Apply a light brown matte shadow just above eye crease.

- Mascara can be used but with caution. Apply only one coat in black and brush out with lash comb for a more natural look. Blondes look more natural in dark brown.

- Facial hair can be filled in where needed with cake eye shadow or brow pencil in the same shade as facial hair. Focus on beards, sideburns and mustache.

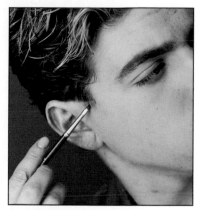

Clean up facial hair

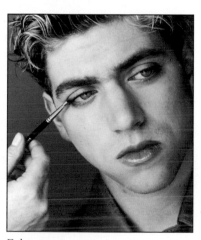

Enhance eyes

TIP

Only use foundation or blemish concealers on the face, not under eye concealers that contain oil and can cause breakouts.

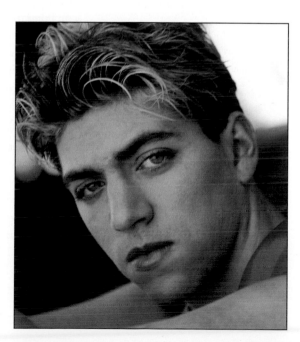

Keep These Notes in Mind: Advice from Judges

- Make sure brows are defined, arched and extended properly, especially for the very fair or those with dark skin tones.

- All ages should have even-looking skin. Use the correct foundation, especially where cheek color is applied to prevent overly flushed faces. Avoid light-reflecting liquid makeup as it makes the face look too fair under stage lights. If foundation looks too light against the body try a darker shade of powder instead of foundation, to look more natural. Powder is a must to avoid excessive shine.

- Eye shadow should look blended and in neutral colors that do not fight with different costume changes. Avoid bright colors like blue, green, or purple.

- Eyeliner should be left open at the outer eye corners so eyes do not look closed and small. Beware of too much black eye liner unless the theme calls for that look, and never on the lower lid ridge.

- Wear false lashes. They do open your eyes!

- Cheek color should be used to flush. Use a contour cheek shade to define features.

- Lip liner should be used with lipstick to shape the lips. Keep sides of lips full for profile views.

- Don't let lips get too dry. Treat your lips regularly.

- Be cautious when using glitter. Apply only to key light-catching points. Never use on male dancers.

- When wearing a hat, especially those with brims that cast shadows, be sure to dress up lips using gloss, glitter or a dramatic lip color.

- When performing a classical ballet or any number that is ethereal, highlight with shimmer powder on cheekbones and eyes. Matte faces look plain and dull.

- When lots of skin is exposed on the back or midriff, add a shimmer lotion or sparkling powder over bare areas. For glitzy costuming, dress up your skin with glitter spray.

- Remember to choose appropriate makeup for the themes of your dances: for the 1940s era use a strong eyeliner on the upper lids with strong lips, for the 1960s use white shadow and white lips or for the 1980s use bright shadow and lips. (For much more about theme and era makeup, see chapter seven, page 103.)

- Makeup for traditional or cultural numbers like clogging, African or Latin should stay with the look of that culture.

- Avoid too many rhinestones. Neck chokers, earrings, bracelets or hair jewels, choose two— and keep it simple.

- Unless it's part of the number, avoid mouthing the words. It's distracting.

- Don't move the music tempo faster than the song is being played. Need a faster tempo? Find one.

- Think about your undergarments. Be sure they match and do not show under or outside of your costume.

- Watch facial expressions. Don't make faces (look strained, with lips puckered). Instead, make eye contact and smile.

- Wear costumes that are secure to avoid embarrassing wardrobe problems.

6
High
Performance Hair

Performers who have costume changes need to change their hair and makeup a bit to go with the theme of each number. This is as important as changing costumes and music. It shows that you have given thought to your total look and adds excitement to your performance. But changing into a new hairstyle can take time—usually there is only enough time for a quick backstage touch-up. The fastest and most effective way for a quick change hairstyle is to use a hairpiece, accessory or wig. This is a common beauty must-have in show business, and now you can learn the secrets to fabulous hair in minutes.

Drawn-on Drama *(Theme Curls, Sideburns & Mustaches)*

LATIN COSTUMES

Latin costumes can have a more romantic feel when a small curl is added at the side of the face for drama. This is a very *Spanish Rose* style and looks great with complimentary costuming. Shakespeare themes also come alive when curls are placed around the forehead and sides of the face.

MASCULINE LOOK

Placing additional hair around the face by drawing on sideburns or a mustache is an easy way to create a masculine look. To get the look: use a wet/dry cake liner or brow pencil in your hair shade. Light blondes should choose a color that is two shades darker than your hair color so the look will show up on stage.

MAKEUP REMOVAL

To remove quickly for the next number, use a non-oily eye makeup remover pad wrapped around a Q-tip and gently swipe away. It should take a few clean swipes and you are ready to go back on stage.

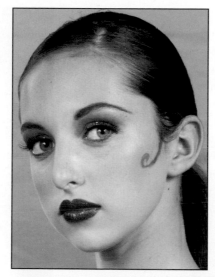

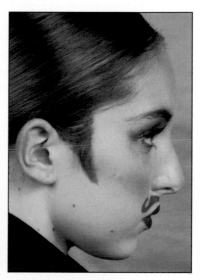

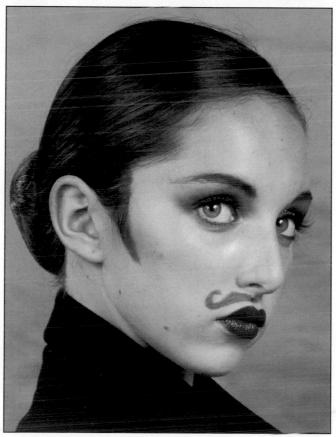

Hairpieces

IT'S A CINCH

Drawstring hairpieces look the most natural. These are secured over hair styled into a bun and lay close to the head. Then place little combs at the top and bottom next to an elastic cinch and secure it around the bun. The cinch can be easily reinforced for more hold by pushing bobby pins into the sides, securing the hairpiece to the bun.

THE FINGER CLIP

Hairpieces with finger clips can work well, especially with long heavy styles. The challenge with this piece is to keep it from sticking out unnaturally and to secure it when you will be moving a lot. The best way to wear this type of hairpiece is to unwrap the hair bun, pull the remaining ponytail up against the head, and secure the hairpiece just above the ponytail elastic band. This will keep the clip closer to your head. Separate the ponytail into two pieces above the hairpiece and wrap each one around each side next to your head, securing at the base of the hairpiece. This will give it a more natural look.

BEAUTIFUL BUNS

For those who want a perfect-looking bun but don't have enough hair or have too many layers in their hair, try bun covers. Just put your hair in a messy bun and pop the cover over the top. They are secured with little built-in combs, an elastic cinch and a few strategically placed bobby pins.

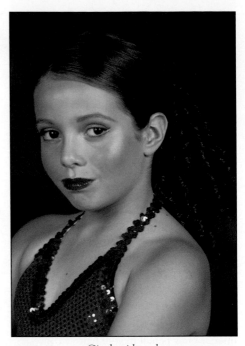

Cinch with curls

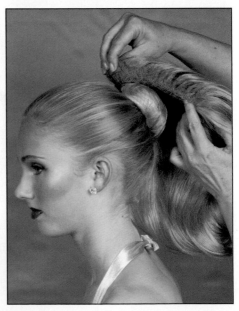

Cinch over bun

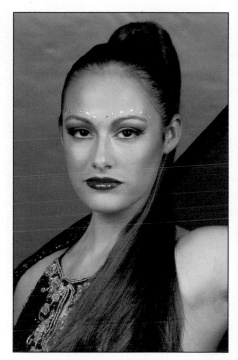
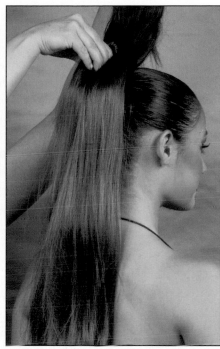

Finger clip pony

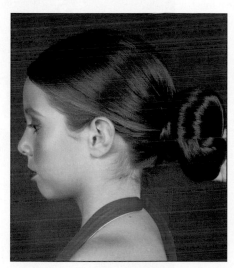
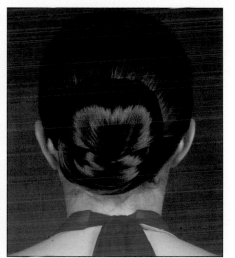

Secure over bun

Hair Accessories

ELASTIC HAIRPIECES

These are elastic bands of hair that are either curly, straight or braided, and come in natural or fun punky bright colors. Wrapped twice around the base of a bun, these can change your look quickly and effortlessly. Mix up the look to go with your performance theme.

RHINESTONES

You can add drama to your hair with rhinestone clips, pony band covers, headbands and mesh bun covers. These add glamour, so be sure the performance or the piece calls for that kind of elegant look. Glue stones to bun covers, combs or hair bands. New "stick on" rhinestone designs, for one-time use, are available. Rhinestones with Velcro® on the back work well in hair. If you love rhinestones, be sure to use no more than two rhinestone accessories at a time. Too many sparkling accessories can be distracting.

HAIR COLORING POMADE

Pomade can add color, shine, controls frizz, and comes in a variety of colors including gold or silver. Scoop out a small amount. Rub between the palms of your hands, then spread through pieces of your hair to create colorful light-catching streaks. Remember, the more you use, the greasier your hair looks, so use it sparingly.

HATS

Hats can add character and drama, but when wearing a hat, be sure your lips have life by using a bit of gloss for shine or glitter for a twinkle. Hats cast shadows on your face, covering your eyes and leaving the focus on your mouth.

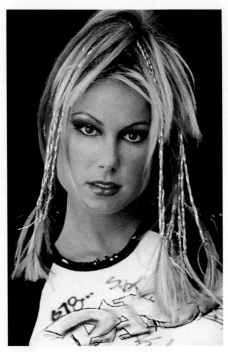

Braided elastic

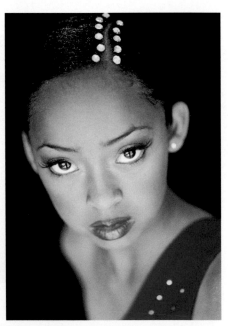

Rhinestones

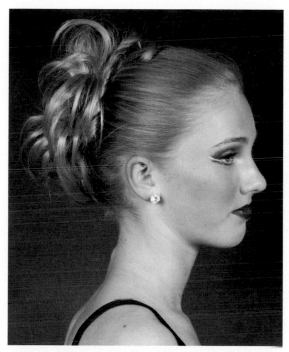

Straight elastic

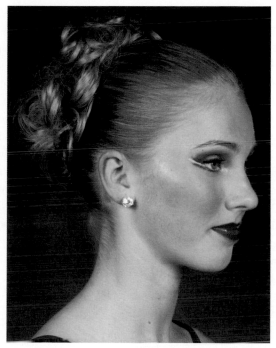

Curly elastic

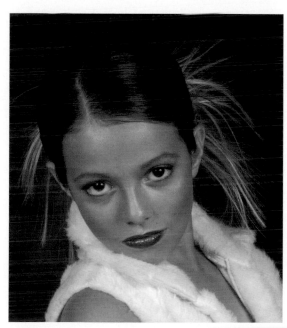

Color elastic

Wigs

Using a wig can be a wonderful way to quickly change your look, creating new excitement and show appeal. Don't be afraid to experiment, but do think through your total look, head to toe. When performing in a group number, uniformity is still very important, even when it comes to hair.

CHOOSING A WIG

Celebrity wigs look natural because they are. Real human hair wigs are very expensive and look fabulous, but on stage, synthetic hair can look just as good. Be sure to buy quality synthetic hair that moves and looks like real hair. A good wig will have the hair sewn into a mesh cap that allows your head to breathe.

CARE FOR A WIG

Wash with gentle shampoo. Also, professional wig shampoos are available. Keep in mind that synthetic wigs are plastic and not real hair. But just like real hair, never brush or style when wet, since the strands are more delicate and break when wet. Comb out only when dry using a wide-toothed comb, working from the ends up. Never use hot styling tools on synthetic hair. They will melt!

PUTTING ON A WIG

When using a wig, be sure to secure it in a professional way. Here's how your favorite stars wig out:

The most natural way to wear a wig is to first part your hair down the middle in the back. Wrap the right side of your hair around your head going forward to the left, then secure at the side and front of your head. Repeat on the right side. Make sure the hair is lying flat against your head. If the wig will be worn for a long time, keep edges and strays in check with a wig cap. Keep the wig secure by using small bobby pins that match the wig hair color. Never secure the edges of the wig around your hairline as these bobby pins are easily noticed. Instead, push bobby pins through the mesh of the wig at the sides (not edges), top and back of your head.

When changing quickly from a bun hairstyle to a wig, unwrap your bun, separate the ponytail into two pieces, and secure each half along sides of head working forward. Keeping the ponytail in place will help you quickly go back to a bun style if needed. Unwrapping the bun prevents a noticeable bump under the wig at the back of the head.

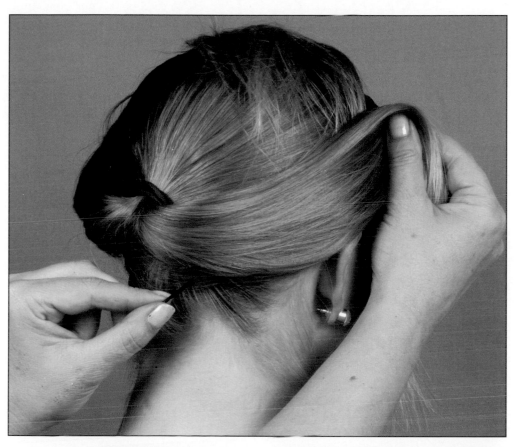

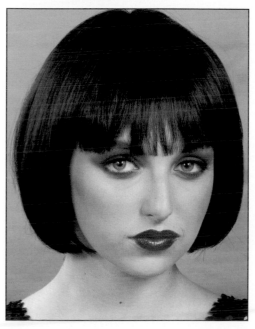

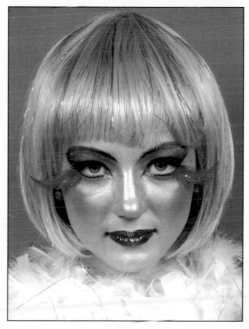

Styling for the Stage

In most performance situations, changing hairstyles can be difficult. There is simply not enough time. That's why most performers prefer hairpieces and wigs. If you are able to keep the same hairstyle throughout your performance but would like a change from the classic bun, here are a few variations that are easy to do and look great.

For a twist on a classic bun, pull hair into a ponytail. Take separate strands of hair and wrap into small buns around the ponytail band. Secure with bobby pins. This looks like clusters of rosebuds when complete. For a funky casual bun, pull hair back into a ponytail, make a bun, leaving the end of your ponytail out of the bun. Secure and drape remaining hair around the sides of the bun.

Rosebud buns around face can be achieved by using tiny rubber bands (safe for hair) to secure small pieces of hair around the face. Three small buns on either side of face should be enough to create nice balance. Secure with small bobby pins. For a funky look, leave the tip of the small ponytail out of the bun. Instead pull it through the bun's center so it sticks up like a spike, and secure the bun.

For those that have difficulty achieving a smooth pulled-back hairstyle, try pulling your hair back while still wet. Use hair gel to smooth down the sides and any stray strands.

7
Stage Makeup in Character Fantasy Faces

Makeup styles change in every era just like fashion does. Creating theme makeup can capture the look and drama of costuming and music, taking the performance to a new level of excitement. To help you create your theme, here is a guideline for several different eras and the makeup that characterizes each one. *(This chapter contains colors, styles and application instructions for the ultimate fantasy look. Other chapters, especially chapter five, will help you with in-depth application techniques, how to determine your skin type and the kinds of products to buy.)*

1920s See Chicago (this chapter)

1940s Strong black liner across upper lid only, sweeping out beyond crease at outer eye corners. Strong thin brows and rich red lips, lined full and round at the sides. Bright red cheek color on the apples of cheeks.

1950s Bold baby blue eye shadow, heavy black eye liner on upper lid that sweeps out and up just beyond eye crease. Bright pink lips and cheeks. Thin brows.

1960s See Groovy Baby (this chapter)

1970s Frosted blue eye shadow on lids and white eye shadow under brows. Pinky cheek color on apples and pale frosted pink or white lipstick. Thin dark brows.

1980s Bright eye shadow in at least three colors. Thick, dark eyebrows, and bright glossy lipstick. Think of Cindy Lauper! Another popular look in this era was bright glossy red lips with dark brown eye shadow or the look of the "Robert Palmer Girls" in the music videos "Addicted to Love" and "Simply Irresistible."

Chicago (1920s flapper)

THE LOOK

In the "Roaring Twenties," fashionable ladies wore smoldering dark eye shadow with strong, smudged eye liner under lower lashes; heavy, defined eyebrows and dark rosebud lips.

HAIR

❶ Depending on the character, choose between platinum white or black wigs in a short bob style.

EYEBROWS

Define, arch and extend brows. Use a brow color in a shade darker than your natural brow. Do not blend—leave brows looking drawn on.

EYES

First prepare eyelid, beginning by dusting it with face powder for a smooth dry surface. For more drama, use a powder with gold shimmers. • Define and create a sultry look by brushing dark brown shadow across entire lid up into crease. With a dry pointed brush, blend dark brown shadow under bottom lashes. • Balance and warm eyes with burgundy eye shadow above crease and across eye bone from the beginning of brow to the end. • Highlight brow arch and pull lid forward at the center with a cream color shimmer eye shadow. • Line eyes with wet black cake liner across three-quarters of the upper lid, then use dry liner over brown shadow under lower lashes so it looks smudged. Leave eye corners open. Use white eye pencil to line between the upper and lower liners and on lower eyelid ridge. For more glitz, apply a little silver glitter to the center of eyelids.

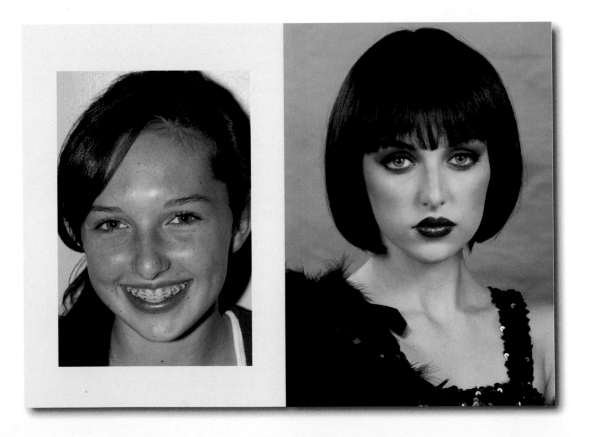

THE CANVAS

Clean up eye shadow flecks from under the eyes and apply foundation, using downward strokes, over face and slightly onto throat. Use concealer to cover dark under eye circles. False lashes enhance this look. Use thick black lashes trimmed to fit your eyes and apply one coat of mascara to top and bottom lashes.

LIPS

❷ Fill in lips with deep burgundy lip pencil. Line lips small at the sides and full at the top. Brush on a rich deep burgundy lipstick and blend into lip pencil. Pop center of lips with a glossy shimmer.

ADD COLOR

Flush apples of cheeks and temples with a red/burgundy cheek color.

❸ With this same color, using a pointy liner brush, apply over eyeliner at the center of bottom lashes. Use sparingly.

GLAMOUR

Dust cheekbones, chest and shoulder with gold sparkling powder.

❶

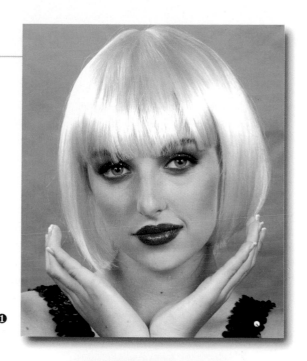

❷

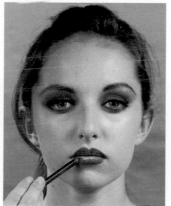

❸

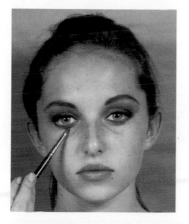

Groovy Baby (1960s)

THE LOOK

For a style of the mod 60s choose groovy dark eye shadow in black highlighted with white shimmer. Accentuate with thick black false lashes and pair with white or light beige lip color.

HAIR

A high ponytail with a lift at the crown, a flip at the jaw line and a stick-straight part down the middle. Headbands can be worn with hair down—keep a high lift at the crown and flip at the shoulders —or wear a pageboy satin hat.

EYES

To highlight the eyes, apply white matte shadow all over eyelid. For glamour use a white shimmer powder. Be sure to apply at inner eye corners. To define, use a matte black or gray shadow just above eye crease from the inside, blending across crease, sweeping up at the outer side toward the end of brow. Line the eyes with wet black or gray eye shadow, using the tip of a pointed brush dipped in eyeliner sealer or water. Stir to create a liquid and line across lid. Leave inner corner of eye open. Apply across lid extending up and out, stopping just above crease at outer eye corner. Create a thin line under bottom lashes. Do not blend eye liner. Use white eye pencil on lower eyelid ridge and between the two lines at the outer eye corners. Apply thick, long black false lashes cut to fit your eye. Finish with two coats of mascara on top and bottom lashes. Clean up under-the-eye mess.

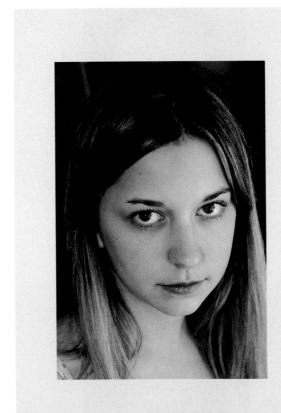
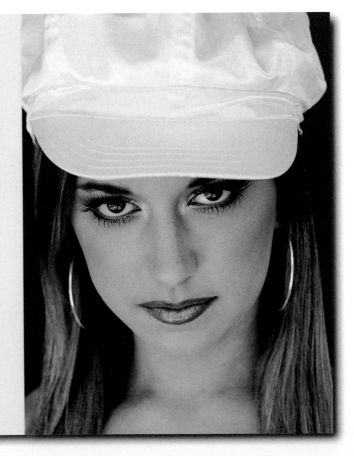

THE CANVAS

Apply foundation, concealer and powder to even skin tone.

LIPS

Blend a natural lip pencil in a brown tone on lips. Leave just the center of the upper and lower lip pencil-free. Apply a light shimmer lipstick in white/pink or white/beige (shown). For the ultimate full lips, use a high-shine lip gloss. Try a white/silvery color just in the center of lips.

BROWS

Make brows as thin and defined as possible with a high arch at the center. To make thin brows, cover outer edges with white pencil or foundation. To create a higher brow arch, apply a small amount of white shimmer shadow just below it.

CHEEKS

Define facial features with a natural pink/beige cheek color, under cheek-bones and along sides of nose. Flush cheeks with pink, if needed. Enhance cheekbones with a white sparkling face powder high up on the bone.

GLAMOUR

Glitter can enhance the glamour of this look. Apply thinly across the lash line and on lips. Blue brings out this costume and white opal on the lips sets the tone of the mod era. ❶ For sparkling hair, spray it with glitter spray for sparkling locks.

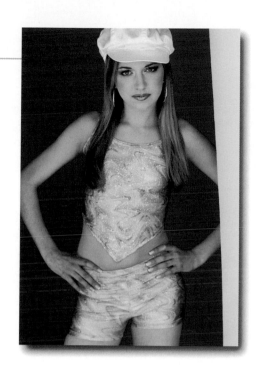

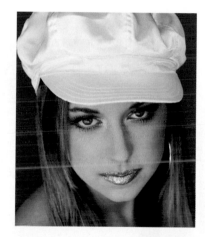

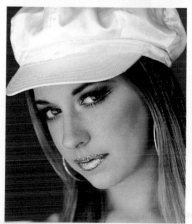

❶

TIP

When wearing a hat that has a brim, be sure to enhance lips with some glitter or gloss, as shadows from the brim wash out lip color.

All That Jazz

THE LOOK

This is the vamp. A look designed for dramatic stage lighting. Bold lip and eye color are essential as the face can become lost under a top hat. Add fishnets and a cane to complete the look.

HAIR

Hair is pulled back in a low ponytail or bun so a top hat fits well.

BROWS

Define and extend out a bit further than your natural brow line.

EYES

Set eyelid with face powder. For smoky eyes, blend matte, dark plum/purple eye shadow above crease onto eye bone. Blend from outer edge of eye to about three-quarters of the way across. • To balance and brighten eyes, apply matte burgundy eye shadow across eye bone. • To highlight eyes, apply sparkling silver eye shadow into inner half of lid, and beneath brow. • Line under lower lashes using burgundy eye shadow with a liner brush dipped into water or eyeliner sealer. Soften line with a Q-tip or dry brush to create a smudged look. Repeat using black eye shadow and apply to outer half of upper eyelid, sweeping line up into crease. • For open, bright eyes apply bold, full false lashes, then add one coat of mascara to top and bottom lashes.

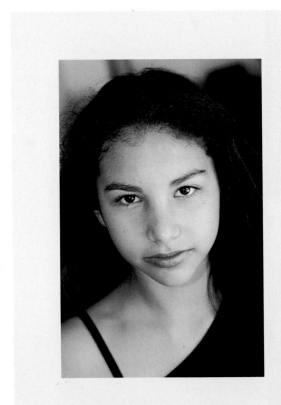
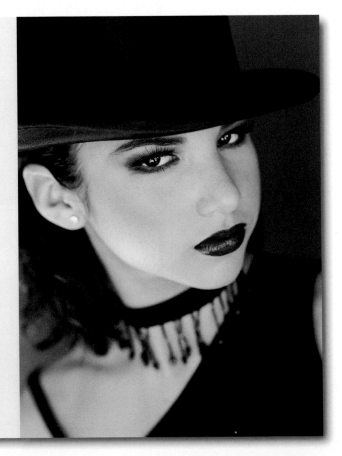

THE CANVAS

Apply foundation and concealer; set with powder.

LIPS

Line lips with dark burgundy lip pencil. Apply to entire lip. Use a deep, rich burgundy lipstick over lip pencil and finish with clear lip gloss for a mega shine.

CHEEKS

Contour the face by defining cheekbones and sides of nose with pink/brown contour cheek color. Use red blush on apples of cheeks.

GLAMOUR

Add drama with glitter along lash line in subtle purple. ❶ For a glitter flash with the look of diamonds, try a little silver glitter on lips, eyes and cheekbones.

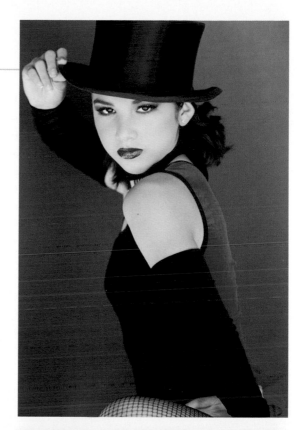

TIP

When using strong colors, make sure to blend one color into the edges of another for a more polished look.

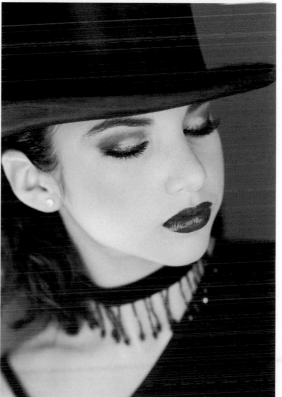

❶

Orchid Fairy

THE LOOK

Whimsical twinkling fairies. The perfect theme for soft, sweet, pastel costuming.

BROWS

Arch and extend brows for a polished frame to the eyes.

HAIR

Up in a bun, with a soft side part. Rhinestones are scattered through the hair to catch light, and delicate lilac orchids are at the crown.

EYES

Set eyelid and define eyes using dark plum shadow. Blend halfway across lid, and finish just above crease, parallel to the end of eyebrows. • Create balance and warmth to eyes with pink/burgundy eye shadow applied just above crease, three-quarters of the way across eye bone. • Highlight and create sparkling eyes with white shimmery shadow under brow, across inner half of eyelid and at inner corner of eyes. • Stir the plum shadow with a pointed brush wet with water or eye liner sealer. Line outer half of upper lid and outer half of lower lid. To keep eyes open do not meet liners at corners of the eye. Use white eye pencil between the two lines at the outer eye corners. Clean up under eyes. • Cut false lashes to your natural length and apply. Apply one coat of mascara to top and bottom lashes.

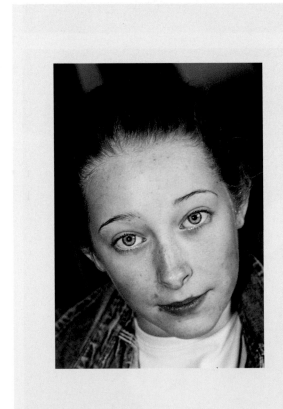

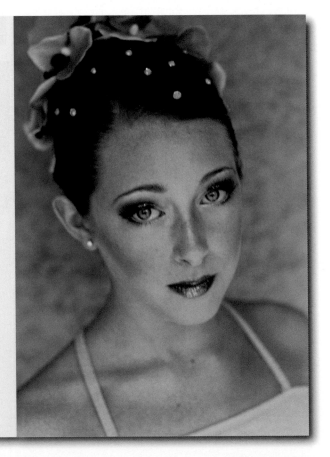

THE CANVAS

Even skin tone with foundation and concealer; set with face powder.

CHEEKS

Define cheekbones and nose line with a pink/brown cheek color. Sweep a bright pink blush on the apples of the cheeks. Enhance cheekbones with a silvery shimmer powder.

LIPS

Define lips using a pink/brown lip pencil. Apply over most of lip, leaving the inner lip free. Use creamy lipstick in a sparkling medium pink shade. For large stages use sheer burgundy and highlight center of lips with shimmery white lipstick.

GLITTER

Create fantasy with twinkles from pastel or opal glitter. Seal on cheek bones, eyelids and lips. Spray hair and body with glitter to add twinkle and magic.

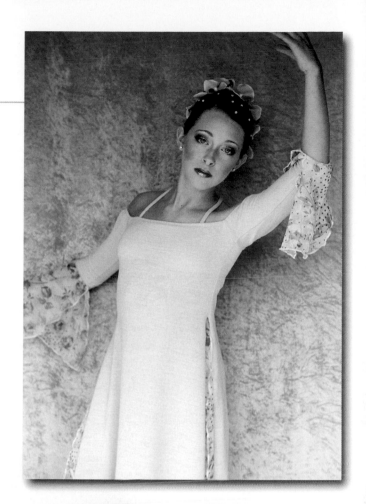

TIP

Buy imitation flowers at the local craft store. Pop off the plastic stems. Push a bobby pin around base of the flower and secure around bun.

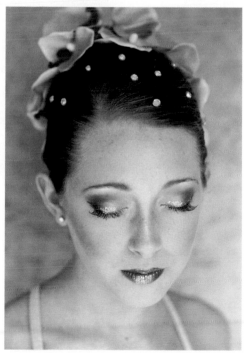

Cats

THE LOOK

For purr-fectly beautiful cat makeup, the most important tool is your imagination. Create a tiger cat using black, white, brown, red/orange and gold. For a lion face, use black, white and gray colors. For a leopard, try adding spots. The key is to layer colors like stripes on a cat's coat. The more layers that show, the more the colors look like fur. • *Tools:* Stage-pigmented eye shadow colors used wet or soft colored face/eye pencils or grease paint in white, red/orange, yellow, brown, and black.

HAIR

Create ears by taking the front portion of your hair, parted down the middle, into two sections. Twist each section around into a circle and run the tip through the center so it stands straight up. Use bobby pins to secure.

THE CANVAS

Even out skin by applying foundation over face and onto throat. Use concealer under eyes to lighten dark circles.
• Highlight using a white pencil. Stroke color onto center of forehead, down center of nose, under brows, around upper lip (to create a muzzle) on chin and high on cheekbones.
• Define features with black pencil or wet/dry eye shadow cake: apply to brows, sweeping up to create stripes, use as eye liner to shape cat eyes (up at outer eye corners and down into inner eye corners), define tip of nose down to the upper lip and over middle of chin. Last, add spots for whiskers. (A liquid liner is great for whiskers too.)❶

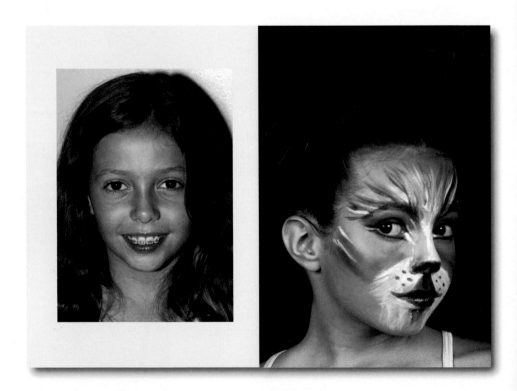

EYES

Set foundation and lids with sheer face powder. Contour crease with dark brown eye shadow. Apply wet with a pointy brush alternating black and white stripes from brows. Lift and warm eyes with red/brown eye shadow onto eye bone.❷ Highlight eyes with gold/yellow eye shadow on inner lid and under brow. Apply white eye pencil onto inner eye corners between liners.❸ Apply false lashes and one coat of mascara to top and bottom lashes.

CONTOURS

Contour features with dark brown blush. Stroke a few black, brown and white stripes along sides of face for definition.❹ Define nose with brown eye shadow or blended eye pencil.❺

LIPS

Lips should look small and thin. Apply brown or black pencil or eye shadow onto inner lip and smudge in. Create a cat smile by sweeping color out and up at sides of mouth. Enhance lips with red/ brown lipstick if needed.

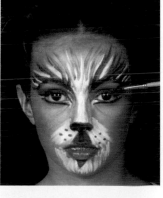 ❶

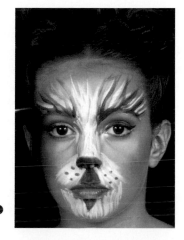 ❷

❸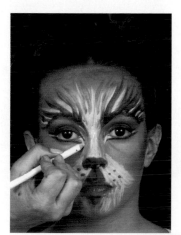

❹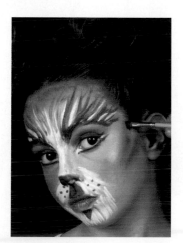

❺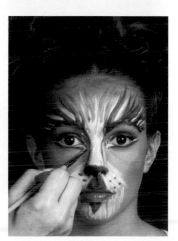

Hip Hop

THE LOOK

The focus is on dark bold eyes and very glossy shimmer lips. It is more of an edgy street look to go with the strong, powerful and modern sounds of rap or hip hop.

HAIR

Funky street hair. Put a straight spikey hairband around bun or add a band of braids (shown). Try different spikey add-on hair colors for a punk look, or wear a baseball hat backwards to allow your face to show.

EYES

Set eyelid with face powder. To define the eyes, blend matte black eye shadow across lid and up just above the crease. Extend out toward the end of eyebrow. • To balance and tone down the black, blend in edges using a peach or light brown eye shadow across eye bone. • Create a wet shimmer effect on center of lid, inner eye corner and under brow arch with a sparkling white shimmer powder or eye shadow. For more glitz apply silver glitter onto center of eyelid. Intensify eyes by lining with black shadow with a pointed liner brush. By not wetting the black eye shadow, a more smudged eye line can be achieved. Be sure not to let top and bottom liner lines meet at the corners. Apply white eye pencil between the two lines at the outer eye corners and on the lower lid ridge to keep the eyes open. • Apply lots of black mascara or false lashes to bring out eyes.

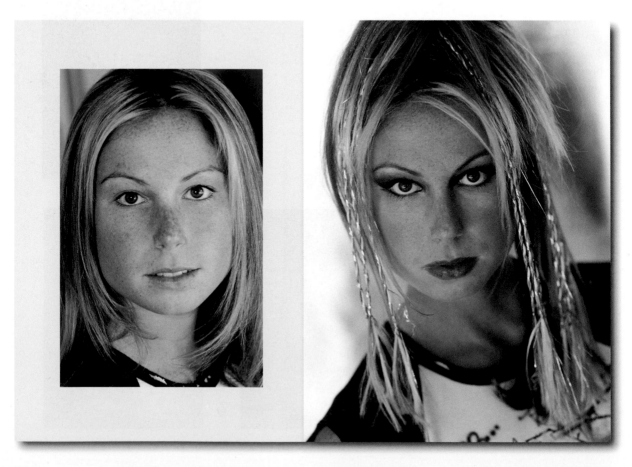

THE CANVAS

Even skin tone with foundation, concealer and set with powder.

CHEEKS

Contour cheekbones and sides of nose with a pink/brown cheek color. Add a little color to the apples of the cheeks, temples and forehead in a peachy cheek shade.

BROWS

Frame eyes by shaping and lengthening brows. Keep them thin.

LIPS

Line with pink/brown natural-looking lip pencil. Brighten with a creamy peach lipstick and add sparkling gold or silver super-shine lip gloss.

GLAMOUR

Enhance features with shimmering sheer face powder on cheekbones, down center of nose, on throat, chest and shoulders.

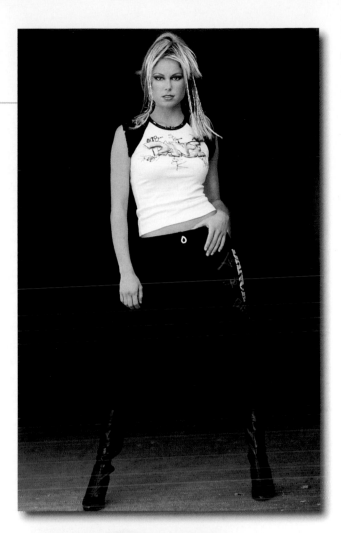

TIPS

If you are going from red lipstick worn in another number to this look, blot the lips and apply peach-colored lipstick or a light shimmer lipstick, then gloss over it. Just be sure to tone down the red color, as it does not go well with this street look.

For more drama, apply glitter on the center of eyelids.

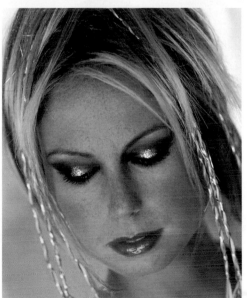

Desert Princess

THE LOOK

A Mediterranean costume with lots of twinkling jewels and beading. A flowing scarf to move around face and body. Exotic, lined cat eyes and rich lips.

HAIR

Think of a genie; a high, long, straight ponytail with a braid or another ponytail wrapped around the base.

BROWS

Shape with brow cake or pencil extending outer ends. Avoid a downward slope.

FLAWLESS SKIN

Use oil-free moisturizer to stay fresh. Clean up fallen eye shadow. Even skin tone with oil-free foundation and concealer. Set with translucent face powder.

EYES

Set lids with face powder for a matte finish.❶ Define with black matte shadow, starting at outer eye corner stopping just above eye crease facing toward the end of eyebrow.❷ Continue to define the crease above the eye across the eye bone. Balance eyes to lips with terracotta matte eye shadow on eye bone from end of eyebrow to its beginning.❸ Highlight lid and below brow with cream shimmer eye shadow.❹❺ Line eyes with black wet/dry shadow cake liner across upper eyelid. Sweep down into inner eye corner like a cat's eye and out at the end of eye above crease toward the end of eyebrow. Line lower lash line into inner eye corner and extend out stopping above eye crease parallel to the end of eyebrow.❻ Create pop by using a white shimmer powder at inner eye corner, brow arch and down center of eyelid. Apply thick black false lashes cut to fit.

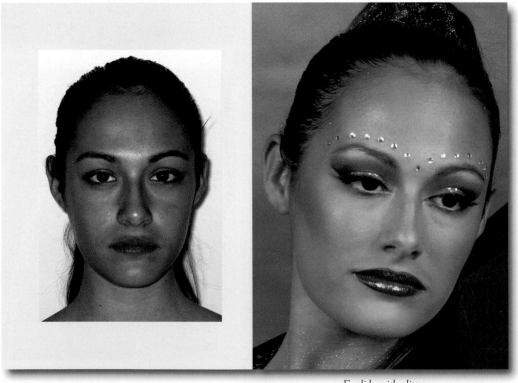

Eyelids with glitter

LIPS

Line with deep burgundy lip liner and add color with deep burgundy red lipstick. Apply thick black false lashes cut to fit.

CHEEKS

Define cheekbones and along sides of nose with a contour shade and flush cheeks with a burgundy red cheek color.

RHINESTONES

To add more glamour and excitement to the face, make a design with rhinestones. Start by creating the design with dots using a black pencil or liner. Squeeze out small drops of lash glue or spirit gum, onto dots, three at a time. Using tweezers, pick up rhinestones and position on top of dots and glue. Allow them to set for a few minutes.❼

GLITTER

Glamorous glitter on lips, eyes, hair and body enhance the glimmer in the costume. Catch lights with complimentary glitter (gold shown) patted on lips and sealed on eyes. Use glitter spray on hair and body to draw attention to skin and form.

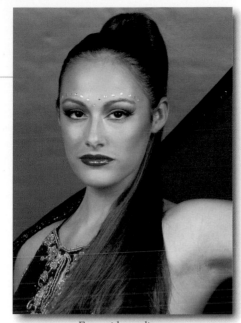

Eyes without glitter

TIP

Rhinestone designs are great for many theme looks including showgirls and jazz numbers.

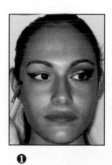 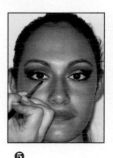 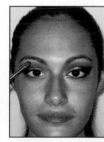 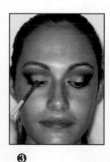 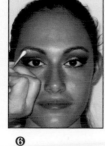 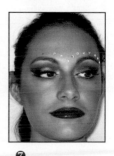 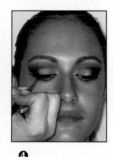

❶ ❷ ❸ ❹

❺ ❻ ❼

Cirque

THE LOOK

A fantasy face with dramatic twinkling eyes and lips. Eyes are framed with thick false lashes on upper lid and feathers sweeping out from lower lid to compliment the feather boa and sparkling multi-colored wig.

HAIR

Slicked back with a side part and low ponytail. To create an out-of-this-world fantasy, wear a platinum bob sparkling with multi-colored tinsel to catch light and add drama. ❶

iEYES

Apply black wet/dry cake eye shadow liner sweeping up toward end of brow, rounding into it, across the center and finishing sweeping down toward sides of nose.❸ Line eyes across eyelid and sweep end of liner into inner eye corner toward side of nose.❹ Define eyes with black matte eye shadow across lid, finishing up slightly above eye crease. Apply red cheek color at the outer rounded lined area of brow bone and under brow, across line, toward the sides of nose. Lashes on the upper lid should be dramatic and black cut to fit. Feather lashes should be applied on outer lower lash line sweeping out. Glitter, in multi-colored pastel sparkles sealed onto outer brow bone and inner eye corners, creates ethereal glamour.

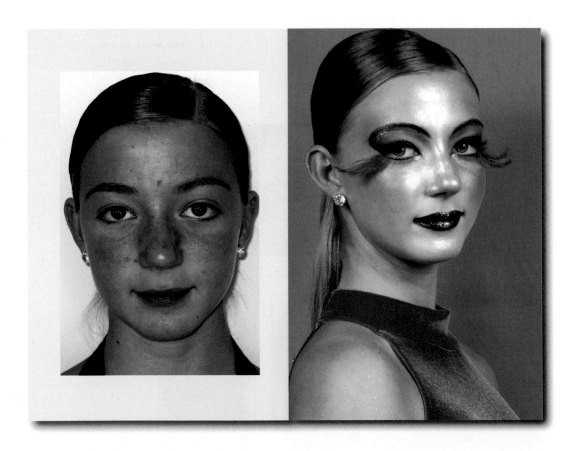

FACE

Prepare face with foundation, concealer and powder. Remember that light shimmer pulls the features forward and matte dark pulls in. White shimmer down the front of the face creates facial features that look out-of-this-world—and more like an exotic creature.❷

CHEEKS

Flush with red cheek color just on apples.

LIPS

Apply red or rich pink lip liner and blend onto lip. Enhance with red or rich pink lipstick. Glitz the lips with fuchsia lip glitter all over lips, then multi-colored opal glitter down the center of lips for pop.

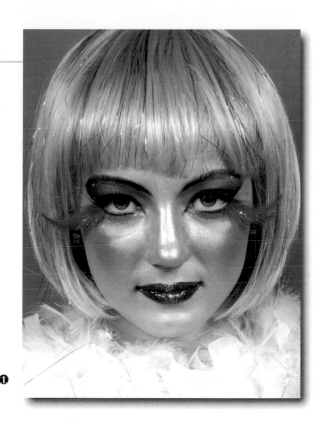

❶

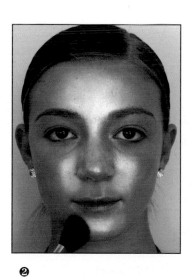

❷

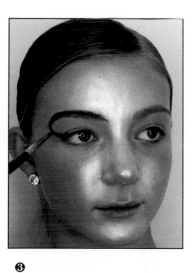

❸

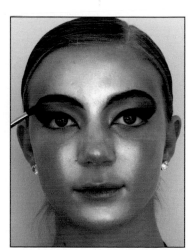

❹

Conclusion

Beauty is just as important as choosing the right music, learning your steps and wearing the right costume. Beauty is more than makeup colors and how you apply them. True beauty comes from loving yourself enough to take care of your body as well as your mind. Find a balance between stress and relaxation, put your body to the test and make time for some gentle pampering. Be creative with your looks. Use this book as a guideline and inspiration to take yourself to a new level of defining your style. Whenever you get the chance to perform, remember that your beauty onstage comes from the love and inspiration you share with others.

Makeup workshops with Christine Dion are available throughout the United States. For information or questions, contact her through her website at *www.modedion.com*, a full beauty resource for performers. All makeup, hairpieces and wigs used on the models in this book are from the Mode Dion Collection. Information on purchasing these products, training and services are on *modedion.com*.